for me. Hope you like it.
thanks again.

REAL ANSWERS
SCIENCE-BASED SOLUTIONS
HEALTHIER SLEEP

smarter sleep

Sleep well!

Mark T. Brown, MD

Old Wives Tales Publishing
Austin, Texas

Created by: Mark T. Brown, MD
Published by: Old Wives Tales Publishing
smartersleep.org
Printed by CreateSpace, An Amazon.com Company

This book is intended to provide medical information, not
diagnose or treat medical conditions. Any and all medical
treatment should be initiated and coordinated by your doctor.

Brown, MD, Mark T.
  Smarter Sleep: Real Answers, Science-Based Solutions,
  Healthier Sleep
ISBN-13: 978-0692480571
ISBN-10: 0692480579
248 pages, plus index.

Available from Amazon.com, CreateSpace.com, and other
retail outlets

Old Wives Tales, Inc.
Austin, Texas

Table of Contents

Forward   v

What is Sleep Medicine?   vi

Acknowledgements   viii

Section 1: Normal Sleep
    Chapter 1: What is Sleep?   2
    Chapter 2: Advice for Smarter Sleep   6

Section 2: Sleeplessness
    Chapter 3: Insomnia   17

Section 3: Snoring and Apnea
    Chapter 4: Snoring   37
        Non-operative treatments   39
        Surgical treatments   42
    Chapter 5: Obstructive Sleep Apnea   51
        Definition   51
        Diagnosis   61
        Treatment   68
            Non-surgical   68
            Surgical   80
        The reality of CPAP   95
    Chapter 6: Central Sleep Apnea   99

Section 4: Sleep Timing Problems
    Chapter 7: Circadian Rhythm Disorders   105

Section 5: Odd Sleep Behaviors
    Chapter 8: The Arousal. Parasomnias   119
    or "Things That Go Weird in the Night."
    Chapter 9: Movements That Wake
    You Up: (A.K.A Dancin' the Watusi)   127
    Chapter 10: Hallucination Parasomnias
    or "What the…"   131
    Chapter 11: REM Associated Parasomnias   133

Chapter 12: Bedwetting   137

Section 6: Excessive Sleepiness
        Chapter 13: Narcolepsy and the
        Hypersomnias (Dig that funky sound)   140

Section 7: Sleep, the Body, and the Mind
        Chapter 14: Medical Problems and Sleep   149
        Chapter 15: Psychiatric Problems and Sleep 169
        Chapter 16: Normal Aging and Changes
        in Sleep   178

Section 8: Pills and Potions
        Chapter 17: Medications and Sleep   184
        Chapter 18: Complementary and Alternative
        Medicines (CAM) and Treatments   201
        Chapter 19: Crazy Quackery and Sleep   208

Section 9: The Technical Discussion
        Chapter 20: The Science of Sleep, 101   216

References   225

Index

Forward

So why write this book? Because I couldn't find one out there for non-physicians that was accessible and intelligent and comprehensive. There is a growing sleep problem in this country. More and more people are diagnosed with Sleep Apnea every day. We are finding increasingly strong links between sleep deprivation and diseases like diabetes and heart problems. Obesity and sleep deprivation have a reciprocal relationship. The 24-hour world we live in seems to make sleep an afterthought. As a society, we don't respect the need for adequate rest. As a result, people are suffering. Fortunately, there is a growing awareness in the medical community of the threats that inadequate sleep pose to personal and public health.

And why should you read this book? An interested person needs to have access to accurate information to make good decisions about sleep and health. I want Smarter Sleep to be a place where you can ask questions and find truthful answers. I intend to cut through the clutter of search engines and medicalese to bring you useful guidance through the strange, surprising and sometimes frightening world of sleep. And maybe when you read it you can get help, or better yet help yourself, to sleep better, be healthier, and be happier. Big goals, I know.

So I hope that you enjoy the read. If you have any recommendations, suggestions, or critiques, let me know. Drop me a line at author@smartersleep.org with whatever feedback you think might help.

What is Sleep Medicine?

If "Sleep Medicine" sounds made up, you are partially correct. I prefer to think of this field as a cobbled-together somewhat organized mess of people who treat sleep disorders. How did we get here? Read on...

In the 1970s increased interest in sleep and sleep biology led to an uptick in research and publishing. Stanford University is credited with having the first academic center to study Narcolepsy. In fact much of the pioneering work in Sleep Medicine came from Palo Alto. (http://sleep.stanford.edu/about/history.html) From there, interest in and awareness of sleep disorders has grown.

The first formalized fellowship training programs were recognized in 1989. The first catalogue of sleep problems was published in 1990. The International Classification of Sleep Disorders first edition, ICSD-1, is now in its 3rd iteration. This landmark book provides consistency, continuity, and updated information about sleep diagnoses and treatments. The American Board of Sleep Medicine (http://www.absm.org) and the National Sleep Foundation (http://sleepfoundation.org) were founded in 1991. The modern structure of Sleep Medicine training and quality assurance has arisen from these organizations. Formal and accredited Board Certification in Sleep Medicine for physicians followed in 2007.

To apply for any board certification, a doctor must be educated and trained in his or her chosen field. They must then provide proof of training and submit to testing, which provides assurance of competency. For Sleep Medicine, the candidate must already be board certified in one of these primary specialties: Neurology, Otolaryngology – Head and Neck Surgery (ENT), Internal Medicine (which also includes Cardiology and Pulmonary Medicine specialists), Pediatrics, or Anesthesia. (Now you see why I said were we a cobbled together bunch.) All of these fields deal with sleep at some level. Sleep Medicine is a subspecialty board within each primary field.

The American Board of Sleep Medicine examination is an 8- hour, comprehensive assessment of a candidate's knowledge about normal and abnormal sleep. Until 2011 docs who could demonstrate that they were practicing Sleep Medicine, fellowship training or not, were able to sit for the exam. Now a formal one-year fellowship at an accredited sleep program is required to take the test.

So when you read through this book and see me refer to a "sleep doctor," in your own mind insert whichever specialist (Neurologist, ENT, Internist, Cardiologist, Pulmonologist, Pediatrician, or Anesthesiologist) you prefer. We each come to the table with our own perspective and skill set. If you need surgery, a Neurologist won't be able to help you. If you have epilepsy, your ENT won't do you much good. But, in the end, we all end up working together to help you to sleep well.

Acknowledgements

Rarely can one person can take all of the credit for a creation. There are teachers and students and occurrences and mistakes and victories and failures and inspirations and desperations and all sorts of experiences that shape what we become. This book is all that and more.

I have had great guidance and editing from my wife, Dr. Ari Brown who is a successful author in her own right. She has motivated me and inspired me to do more and be better. Without her guidance this book wouldn't exist. She is my compass and confidant and will be so forever.

Many other people, knowingly or not, have brought me to this point. Teachers, friends, and family have all helped and supported me throughout my life, providing me with examples of succeeding with grace and excellence.

There are also people who were instrumental in this moment of my life. Their assistance made this book immeasurably better than I could have done on my own. A number of physicians and dentists whose opinions I greatly respect offered guidance and critique: Boyd Gillepsie, MD (Medical University of South Carolina), Nina Shapiro, MD (UCLA, Geffen School of Medicine), Kasey Li, DDS, MD (Stanford Sleep Disorders Clinic), Jay Rubinstein, MD, PhD (University of Washington School of Medicine), Matt Steinberg, DDS (Austin, Texas), and Paige Peterson, PhD, AuD (Austin, Texas). They are all esteemed academicians and clinicians who took their valuable time to review the manuscript and offer insightful comments that made a huge difference. Being challenged by your peers to defend your work always makes it better.

A couple of lay people, who happen also to be sleep patients, were kind enough to give this book a look. Mark Hulak (Seattle, Washington) and a mysterious unnamed local academician (and my patient) provided perspective from the other side of the doctor patient relationship. They both spent an inordinate amount of time helping me with suggestions both contextually and grammatically.

I also need to thank my medical illustrator, Julia Argent. Her line drawings describe and clarify what can be complex anatomical and surgical ideas. Her work makes this a much more approachable tome.

Finally, I have to thank my office. My partner and staff have frequently and patiently waited for me to finish something on this book before they could get me to get back to work again. And I especially thank my right hand and brain, Angelica Rodriguez, soon to be nurse, who keeps me on the right track and makes sure I don't miss dotting any "I's" or crossing any "T's." Her knowledge and ability make me a better doctor.

Section 1: Normal Sleep

"There is a time for many words, and there is also a time for sleep."
Homer, *The Odyssey*

Chapter 1: What is Sleep?

Sleep is this incredible, wonderful, complicated, complex, critical event that occurs every night in your own bed, and you don't even notice – except perhaps for the dreaming part. We should spend about one-third of our lives asleep. And while breathing, drinking, and eating get top billing, sleep is also critical for survival. Without it, we die. Really. And yet, sleep is often considered a necessary evil; just a box to check so we can get on to the more important things in life. Unfortunately, there is a real lack of understanding and insight into the significance of a good night of sleep. And that gives sleep doctors like me a lot to do.

When done right, sleep makes a huge difference in our lives. At night, we are supposed to dial it down and shift to rest, recovery, and renewal mode. Metabolism and bodily functions are coordinated with dark and light so that by the morning we are recharged and ready to get to it again. Timing and quantity of sleep are critical to being healthy. So when sleep goes wrong, it really is a big deal. And sleep issues are surprisingly common.

Some sleep problems are self-induced. Many people sleep too little because they have more important things to do, like watch Late Night or catch the last quarter of Monday Night Football.

Some people have trouble, not of their own making. They can't get to, or stay, asleep. They experience weird sleep activities that disrupt them and/or their bed partners. Some have problems with the regulation, coordination, and/or timing of sleep. Medical and psychiatric problems influence sleep, and vice versa. Medications, prescribed and otherwise, can impact the quality and quantity of sleep.

Before getting to any sleep disorders, it helps to learn about how sleep is supposed to happen. When normal is understood, abnormal sleep and solutions make more sense. So here we go.

Normal Sleep

Sleep is not just about turning off at night and then turning back on again in the morning. It is a very complicated process that is, for the most part, all about the brain. A sleeping brain is a busy brain. It has a long list of required nighttime activities to accomplish in preparation for the next day. This complicated and poorly understood process clears the mind, consolidates memories, and recharges the brain. There is a lot going on up there while the lights are off.

During a normal night, the brain goes through four stages of sleep, cleverly named Stage 1, Stage 2, Stage 3, and REM (REM stands for Rapid Eye Movement, not the alternative 80's rock band). Sleep gets deeper as you progress through Stages 1, 2, and 3. You spend about three quarters or more of the night in these calm, restful periods. The rest of your sleep is REM or "dream" sleep.

You must go through all of the sleep stages in correct order and proportion to achieve a normal, healthy night's sleep. The brain cycles through these stages consistently and methodically during good sleep. Why this pattern is so important, is uncertain. But, without it we don't get quality sleep. In other words, if you don't complete these stages during the night, you will not be at your best during the day.

Stages of Sleep

- Stage 1 sleep occurs mainly at the beginning of the night. Healthy sleepers transition back and forth from Stage 1 sleep to semi-wakefulness as an entrée into to deeper sleep. In Stage1 you are easily awakened. If you do wake up you feel relatively alert and aware. And while it looks kind of creepy, it's normal for your eyes to roll around in your head during this phase. (Watch a baby fall asleep in your arms sometime to witness this Exorcist-like moment.) Only about 10% of the night is spent in this stage. Problems in Stage 1 can lead to "sleep onset" Insomnia. Instead of the normal back and forth of awake and asleep, insomniacs have more periods of being awake and struggle to move into deeper sleep.

- Stage 2 is deeper sleep. While it isn't the most restful or critical sleep phase, Stage 2 does help the transition into the deeper stages of sleep. Once you are here you are really and solidly asleep but can still be awakened fairly easily. You spend up to half of the night in Stage 2.

- Deep/Slow Wave Sleep, or Stage 3 sleep, is very important for daily restoration. Healing and repair occur mainly in this deepest

3

sleep. Because Stage 3 sleep is so profound, it is very difficult to awaken from, like waking the dead. Loud sounds, bright lights, or even some physical shaking may be required. And if you do awaken it takes some time to clear away the cobwebs. In Stage 3 we breathe less deeply and frequently. Our hearts beat more slowly. Deep Sleep is what resting and restoring is all about. It occurs mainly in the first half of the night. Ironically, some unusual sleep problems occur in this stage – confusional arousals (the name says it all), sleep walking, and sleep talking to name a few. We will get back to these in the chapter subtitled "Things that Go Weird in the Night."

Then it all gets crazy in REM…

- REM (Rapid Eye Movement) sleep is totally different compared to the other stages. REM sleep occurs periodically throughout the night, but mostly in the early morning hours. About 15-25% of the night is spent in REM. Your first REM sleep stage may happen in the first hour or two of sleep. Subsequent REM stages become longer and more frequent as the night wears on.

As the name suggests, the eyes move back and forth rapidly during Rapid Eye Movement sleep. Also, the heart beats erratically. Blood pressure goes up and down. Breathing varies tremendously. All the while, your muscles are almost completely inhibited from movement.

REM sleep is the time for dreams, nightmares, memories, and learning. It is here that the majority of those weird stories you tell over breakfast occur. Because movement is inhibited, healthy sleepers cannot act out their dreams. That's good news for people who dream about flying like a superhero. REM sleep disorders can be pretty dangerous! (More on that later.) Nightmares also usually happen in REM sleep.

Amazingly the brain is just as active in REM as it is when you are awake. But, even though the brain is super busy, if you don't get much REM sleep you awaken tired.

Getting rested is only part of the story in REM. This is also the time for your brain to process memories and learn. Fun fact (in case you ever appear on Jeopardy): adults spend 15-25% of their sleep in REM. Newborns spend 50% of their sleep in REM, presumably because babies are all about discovering and learning about the world around them.

While you sleep in REM, you sift through the details of your day, filing away important thoughts and information for later use. Dreams may help relive and make sense of life experiences, preparing them for memory. There are a couple of theories on how this process occurs. Either the brain organizes and stores daily experiences, or sifts through and discards unimportant clutter while we are asleep. Either way, sleep helps organize and categorize information. See? Studying at bedtime before that big test really does help! (Although, studying AND getting a good night's sleep are equally important for getting that A+.)

[If this isn't enough information for you and you really need the scientific answers with the long, convoluted, medical jargon, go to the back of the book in Chapter 20, "The Science of Sleep 101." There you will find a more specific and anatomical explanation of our current understanding about what happens when we are asleep.]

It is amazing to know what went on while you were sawing logs last night. It should give you an appreciation for how complicated the process of sleep really is…and where things can go wrong.

Chapter 2: Advice for Smarter Sleep

"A ruffled mind makes a restless pillow." Charlotte Bronte.

The first rule to remember is this: Sleep is Important. Learn to prioritize it for better health. Not everyone has a sleep problem, but everybody sleeps. Doing it right is not as easy as it may sound. Getting good rest for the sake of your health should be a priority.

There may seem to be so many more important things to do than sleep. Work, family, Monday Night Football; you know, important stuff. Unfortunately, not sleeping enough can lead to significant health and medical problems. It really is <u>that important</u> to get a good, restful night of sleep. Read on for some tips.

Q. What do I need to do to get a good night's sleep?

Okay, this is going to sound pretty simple—because it is. Prioritize sleep. And sleep enough.

There are many distractions that can keep you from getting to bed or keep you from sleeping once you are there. Don't sacrifice sleep to accomplish one more item on your to-do list.

Do you want to perform your best at work? Do you want to be a great Little League coach, and a contributing member at your place of worship, and a loving spouse and parent, and a good friend, and a diehard fan, and well read, and super awesome in all of the other things you do with your life? It helps to be well rested. If you don't get the sleep you need, you are going to be tired. And if you are chronically sleep deprived it is really hard to do all those great things and do them well.

Q. How much sleep do I need?

According to the National Sleep Foundation (**NSF**) adults need 7 to 8 hours of nightly sleep.

Clearly, sleeping too little takes its toll. But you may be surprised to know that sleeping TOO much (9 or more hours) can also be a problem. Some studies show that excessive sleep is associated with health problems. But the jury is still out about whether being a "long sleeper" (sounds like a Seinfeld episode) is actually that dangerous, or whether people with medical problems tend to sleep longer.

Getting that 7 or 8 hours of sleep seems to be just about right for most people.

Q. Everybody else seems to need less sleep than me. If I only sleep 8 hours I feel awful the next day. Why?

Everyone is unique. More than 90% of adults need about 7-8 hours of sleep; others are just naturally long sleepers, healthy and rested on 9 to 10 hours. It's possible that you are in the minority that needs more sleep than the average.

Q. I have never needed that much sleep. I do great on 5 or 6 hours. Am I Superman?

No, you probably aren't a super hero. Either you are one of the very rare "short sleepers," who really are healthy on less than 7 hours a night. Or you are so used to being sleep deprived that you have adjusted and function well enough. I'd suggest you try the Sleep Challenge (see below) to see if you might even do better with more.

Q. What should I do to make sure I am sleeping well?

Read on…

Full disclaimer: the information that follows is a combination of scientific evidence, professional experience, and a dash of common sense. If some of it sounds like what your Mom told you when you were a kid, it's because she was right! (Moms usually are.)

After 20 years of experience in Sleep Medicine I present to you the Top Ten Solutions to the most common sleep problems. If these apply to you, modify your current routine to sleep better.

Top Ten Rules for Good Sleep

1. Have a smart sleep routine. (a.k.a. "Good Sleep Hygiene.")

Mentally preparing for sleep is one of the most important parts of a restful night. The official term for this process is "Sleep Hygiene". No, I'm not talking about your choice of toothpaste or deodorant. Sleep Hygiene refers to the mental and physical wind-down you go through to get ready for bedtime and sleep.

Imagine this scenario: You run three miles, slam down a couple of Doritos® Locos Tacos, and then jump into bed fully dressed without brushing your teeth, washing your face, going to the bathroom, or turning out the lights. Now try to fall asleep. Not a recipe for relaxation, is it? The point is this; you need to prepare for sleep success.

All of us have an ingrained and comforting routine for bedtime. But few people realize how important these nightly rituals are for quality sleep. Putting on your Superman PJs, setting your alarm, and adjusting your pillow are really crucial to settling down for the night. These seemingly mundane activities lay the groundwork for successful and restorative sleep. You aren't really ready to relax and drift off until you have completed your personal routine. Insomnia is often blamed on an inadequate nighttime relaxation routine (A.K.A. Poor Sleep Hygiene).

Look at what you do before you go to bed. See if there are activities counterproductive to relaxation. Discard anything that interferes with the process of unwinding and shedding the worries of the day. That is the best start to a good night's sleep.

2. Follow the Eight Hour Rule.

What time do you go to bed? More importantly what time is your alarm set? Plan on 8 hours between these two events. The math is simple. Following through with this plan? Not so much.

You probably have a predictable, consistent morning schedule. You get up at a certain time every day to get yourself and your family out the door. Sleeping-in is simply not an option.

The variable that most affects the amount of sleep you get, then, is what time you go to bed. Yes, watching your favorite movie again is relaxing, but you may be sacrificing precious sleep time.

So you miss a TV show or sporting event. So what? Set the DVR or check the score in the morning. Staying up late for entertainment will not change your life. But, getting a good night's sleep just might.

Make the choice to go to bed with enough time to sleep 7 to 8 hours and you will feel better, and do better, every day.

3. Comfort is key.

This one may be obvious, but you do need to be comfortable to have a restful night. This doesn't mean you necessarily need to run out and spend thousands of dollars on a new mattress and bedding set; but realize that these are pretty important items in your home. Buying new pillows and sheets every few years, or a new mattress every ten, should be necessity items in your family budget. Good sleep is defined by both quantity and quality. If you aren't comfortable, even if you get 7-8 hours of sleep, you might not fully recharge.

I promise I don't have stock in a mattress company. But, a mattress has a finite life span. If you spend 1/3 of your life lying on something it had better be comfortable. And it will eventually wear out. Caring for your mattress properly can help increase its longevity.

MATTRESS 411

There are four basic types of mattresses: innerspring, airbeds, foam, and latex. Which kind you want with depends on your budget and personal comfort preferences.

In the U.S.,innerspring mattresses are the most popular option. Classically, they are constructed with steel coils underneath for support, and topped with a variety of foam or fiber materials for comfort. Hybrid versions with more comfortable top layers are increasing in popularity. Properly cared for, this type of mattress should serve you well for 8 to 10 years.

Airbeds, like the ones that adjust their firmness to your liking (Sleep Number®) use air-filled chambers instead of steel coils to provide support. Big advantage: you customize your side of the bed making it easier to share a bed with someone with a different firmness preference. Another advantage: airbeds do not form valleys or body impressions (official term "surface distortion") if you sleep in the same position night after night. Airbeds are more expensive than innerspring mattresses, but have a longer life span.

Memory foam mattresses are the longest lasting and are the priciest option of the bunch. Like the other types, foam mattresses offer different levels of firmness. Key advantage: foam material adjusts and conforms to the body and thus reduces pressure points. Downside: foam retains heat making some people feel too hot on them.

Latex (solid foam) mattresses are either made out of synthetic material (petroleum based) or natural rubber latex (for eco-friendly consumers). These mattresses are slightly firmer than memory foam and a bit cooler as well. Be careful of these mattresses if anyone in the house has a latex allergy.

Then there are toppers to provide a soft cushion on top of the mattress. These are additional layers of padding are made of cotton, wool, or gel.

Waterbeds, like Puka beads, were all the rage in the 70's. Today's version is a standard style mattress with water in the center to offer support. If you choose one, just keep the scissors off your bed.

A recent trend is the move toward more "organic" and "natural" products, even in the mattress and bedding you choose. While I can't find a downside in using an "organic" mattress (except to your wallet), I also can't find any scientific evidence to prove their health benefits. First, rarely if ever is an entire mattress truly organic. It may be made with natural materials, but the only reliably and certifiably organic components are cotton and wool used for the fabric coverings. Second, most of the organic mattresses use natural latex foam as the support structure. Most latex is not certified organic.

Health claims for organic mattresses are pretty broad. In fact if you go to some of the organic mattress websites you might think that sleeping on a conventionally manufactured bed is toxic and killing you. There is no scientific evidence for those assertions.

So, if you want an organic mattress and it provides a safe and comfortable place for you to sleep, go for it. If you don't, that's okay too. It is a personal choice, not one backed up by research.

Here is a really useful website that has even more mattress information if you are so inclined.

http://bettersleep.org/mattresses-and-more/

Bottom line: Pick out a mattress type that you can afford and that keeps you comfortable. Make sure that your pillows and mattress are cozy and your sheets are clean and comfy. Then relax in your bed.

4. Your bed is sacred ground.

Do not make the mistake of taking your life to bed with you. We live in a 24/7 world. We are constantly connected to work, our friends and family, the news. The digital age intrudes at every hour. Email and texting, Facebook®, Tumblr®, Instagram®, and whatever else comes next are our constant companions.

But, the bed and bedroom should ONLY be for sleeping and spending time with your significant other. That's it. Really. Your bed is a no-work zone. Remember, you need to have a wind down routine (Sleep Hygeine) that helps you transition from awake and occupied to asleep and resting. Having your laptop and work spread out all over the bed right before you turn out the lights brings the wrong associations to that place and space.

Some people find reading before lights out relaxing. Just make sure it isn't tomorrow's presentation. And avoid computer screens, , and the like. The blue light that comes from them stimulates wakefulness and makes for a poor night of sleep. **(Rahman)** Turn your brain off before bedtime.

5. Set the right temperature.

There is no perfect temperature for sleep. Like the firmness of your mattress and plushness of your pillow, it is all about personal preference. When you share a sleep space, find an acceptable compromise with your sleep partner. The warm-blooded partner may choose to sleep in undies on top of the sheets, while the cool-blooded partner dons thick blankets and fluffy pajamas.

6. Nap wisely.

Naps always sound good, don't they? They are great when you just can't keep your eyes open anymore while reading an office brief or after over-eating your Thanksgiving dinner. At the right time of day and for the proper duration, they can actually do some good. Taking a nap before 3:00PM actually may improve sleep, as long as the nap doesn't last more than hour. However, taking one after dinner (7:00 to 9:00PM) will probably keep you awake at bedtime. Being refreshed after a nap makes it difficult to be sleepy when it is time to turn in for the night. **(Milner)**

And, there is another dark side to napping. New research suggests that people who take naps have a greater risk for Type 2 Diabetes and heart disease. It is unclear what the association is here. As the research unfolds, look for updates.

There is one exception to the "no napping during the day" rule: seniors. Naps really help elderly people stay healthy and mentally sharp. **(Campbell)** Like our canine friends, the elderly are capable of snoozing during the day and sleeping through the night. More on this topic in Chapter 16, Normal Aging and Changes in Sleep.

Bottom line: Naps are fine if they don't keep you up at night. If you need a nap everyday, though, it may be that you are not getting good sleep at night. If that is the case it is probably time to check in with your doctor.

7. Eat Smartly.

Eating within 2 hours of going to bed is a bad idea. A full stomach is not conducive to comfortable sleep. And, if you have heartburn (A.K.A. acid reflux, or "GERD"), eating before bedtime is a particularly poor decision. When food hits the stomach, acid production revs up to start the digestion process. Clearly a belly full of acid is not desirable when you lie down to sleep. Spicy foods are the worst. If you add jalapeños to the stomach acid mix it's going to hurt that much worse when it comes back up. It is hard to focus on relaxing and falling asleep when you are experiencing dinner again, this time mixed with stomach acid.

The take home message is this: avoid a full stomach at bedtime, especially if you are prone to heartburn.

8. Exercise at the right time.

Yes, everyone is busy. It is hard to fit exercise into a daily schedule. And yes, exercise has numerous health benefits; including enabling people to sleep better. Even insomniacs tend to sleep better when they are physically active. The timing of your exercise may impact your sleep.

For most people, exercise is stimulating and invigorating. So, doing it right before bedtime may inhibit relaxation and asleep. Studies show conflicting results, though. **(Youngstedt)** Some of the research supports the common wisdom that physical activity is disruptive to sleep. Other research, in elite athletes, shows just the opposite, even working out within 3 hours of bedtime. **(Myliymaki)**

Most importantly, find time to exercise consistently as part of your overall health strategy. You will have to make your own call on nighttime exercise. If it doesn't bother you and this is the only time you can get to the gym or go for a run, go for it.

9. Caffeinate early (if you must).

Caffeine, as a drug, is a very effective stimulant. And, no matter what the energy supplement commercials say, the invigorating effects of a cup of coffee last up to 5 hours. That is a long time. That cup of cappuccino after dinner out may disrupt your night more than you think, especially if it is not part of your regular routine. If you are used to caffeine in the evening and you sleep well anyway, fine. If not, avoid caffeine after 3pm.

FYI – Both Starbucks® and Ben and Jerry's® coffee ice creams have enough caffeine to disturb sleep too! (See Chapter 17, Medications and Sleep for a list of caffeine offenders.)

10. Drink early (if you so choose).

In the US, alcohol consumption is second only to caffeine in sleep impact. Alcohol, as a drug, is considered a depressant. So, yes, having a drink (or several) can may you feel sleepy. But that is not always a good thing.

Alcohol induces poor quality sleep. After drinking, you may sleep more deeply in the early part of the night but later you don't do so well. Deep slow wave sleep and REM sleep diminishes in the early morning hours as the alcohol wears off. Also, chronic use can lead paradoxically to Insomnia. **(Stein)**

Bottom line: If you choose to have a drink with dinner, cheers! But avoid drinking alcohol right before bed. It will backfire on you. Water, however, makes an excellent nightcap!

THE SLEEP CHALLENGE

Here is where the rubber hits the road. I am going to challenge you to prove to yourself that sleep really is important to good health and well-being. I ask for 1 week of your life, Sunday through Friday. Follow these 10 recommendations and if you are not better rested, more productive, in a better mood, and feeling better in general by the weekend I want to hear about it. Really. Send me an email or letter to let me know what didn't work. If you follow my suggestions I am confident you will understand the power of sleep.

1. **Prepare for bed every night thoughtfully.** Make sure that you have time to wind down for bed every night this week. No last minute disruptions. When it is time to sleep, start getting ready and go!
2. **Follow the Eight Hour Rule**. Every night, go to bed AT LEAST 8 hours before your alarm clock is set to go off. Don't worry this week about what you are missing on TV. Record it and watch on the weekend if you must!
3. **Be cozy in your bed.** Make sure that your mattress is comfortable, the sheets are clean, the pillows are fluffed, and your PJs are pressed.
4. **Your bed is sacred ground**. This is your oasis from the stresses of the day. Sleep and sex and the only 2 activities allowed. Make a conscious effort to leave the day behind before you get ready to sleep.
5. **Keep the room as cool or as warm as you like it.** Find the temperature that is conducive to your sleep and set it. Let your bed partner adjust to your temperature this week if they need to.
6. **Nap wisely.** No naps late in the day. If you catch a little shut-eye, do it before 3 PM and make it short (less than 30 minutes).
7. **Eat smart.** Have the last meal of your day at least two hours before bedtime. Going to bed with a stomach full

14

of food is a recipe for indigestion and Insomnia.

8. **Exercise at the right time:** early in the day. Exercising within an hour of bedtime can be stimulating, not relaxing.

9. **Caffeinate early (if you must).** Caffeine is a stimulant. Avoid having it after 3 PM.

10. **Drink early (if you so choose).** While alcohol makes you sleepy, it also interferes with healthy, regular sleep cycles. No alcohol after dinner. Water is your friend before bed.

Follow these 10 steps every night Sunday through Friday. By Saturday morning, you will be better rested. Honest. And as a result, you will perform better at home and at work and be in a better mood. When you prioritize sleep, you will be happier, healthier and more productive. It just happens.

If you do this Challenge and DO NOT feel better, there is likely more to your sleep problem than not taking care of yourself. Talk to your primary care doctor to make sure that there are no health problems looming that impact sleep.

Section 2: Sleeplessness

Sometimes I lie awake at night, and I ask, "Where have I gone wrong?" Then a voice says to me, "This is going to take more than one night." Charles Schulz

Chapter 3: Insomnia

> When I woke up this morning my girlfriend asked me, 'Did you
> sleep good?' I said 'No, I made a few mistakes.'
>
> Steven Wright

The night before my medical school entrance exam I lay in
bed until about 2:30AM, heart pounding, certain that I was going to
fail because I couldn't sleep. I made it through that test, obviously,
but I have a very vivid memory of how helpless and miserable that
night felt. Everyone has had this happen. Not being able to sleep is
one of life's most frustrating and distressing experiences.

Imagine not being able to sleep EVERY night. Chronic
Insomnia is miserable. There are ways to help.

Q. What is Insomnia?

Literally, Insomnia means "no" (In-) "sleep" (-somnia).
Okay, most of the time people with Insomnia sleep some, they just
have trouble getting there or staying there. One in three American
adults has complained about Insomnia at one time or another. That is
a lot of people! Of those about 100,000,000 people, 10% report
having daytime symptoms (weariness, difficulty concentrating,
fatigue, etc.) due to their restless nights. It takes a significant toll on
our economy, too. An estimated $100,000,000 in productivity is lost
yearly from accidents, hospitalizations, and poor work performance
due to Insomnia. **(Ringdahl)**

**Q. At times I seem to have trouble falling or staying asleep. Does
that mean I have Insomnia?**

No, not necessarily. Everyone has trouble sleeping
occasionally. Insomnia, as a medical diagnosis, is a very specific
condition. You must have all three of the following to meet the
criteria for the diagnosis:

1. **Adequate sleep time.**
   You have to try to sleep and fail. If you voluntarily deprive
   yourself of sleep, you are not an insomniac. If you have

17

enough time in bed to get adequate sleep but you just can't, you may really have it.

2. **No other sleep disorders.**
   No fair claiming Insomnia if you have Sleep Apnea or Narcolepsy or some other sleep problem.

3. **Daytime problems due to lack of sleep.**
   Besides inadequate sleep, you must have at least one of the following consequences: tiredness (fatigue), sleepiness, difficulty concentrating, moodiness, attention or memory problems, proneness to errors or accidents, social or academic performance problems, or continuing concerns and/or worries about sleep. In other words, if you can function well during the daytime you really don't have Insomnia as a diagnosis. That doesn't necessarily mean you are sleeping well. It just means that you sleep well enough not to be a zombie.

Q. How does a doctor diagnose Insomnia?

First, I don't want to blame your sleep problems on Insomnia until we have ruled out anything else that explains your symptoms. Here is the basic rundown of questions:

1. Are you getting enough sleep? When do you go to bed? When do you wake up? What is your bedtime routine? (See Sleep Hygiene in Chapter 2, "Advice for Smarter Sleep.") Setting up healthy sleep habits may be all you need.

2. Do you take naps?
   Naps may interfere with your ability to fall asleep at night. It may be a good idea to discontinue that catnap.

3. Do you take medications or drugs (including caffeine, alcohol, and nicotine) that can disrupt sleep?
   -You may take prescription medications that can affect sleep, which is perfectly fine. But, it might be that by taking these drugs at a different time of the day the effect on sleep can be minimized.

18

-Drugs that don't require a prescription, like caffeine, alcohol, and nicotine, can still impact sleep. If you choose to partake of these, avoid them within a couple of hours of bedtime. (For a more complete discussion go to Chapter 17, Medications and Sleep.)

4. Do you have medical problems that cause pain, frequent urination, or breathing issues?
We need to talk about your health head to toe to be sure to find treatable diagnoses that can improve your sleep. (See Chapter 14, Medical Problems and Sleep for the rundown.)

5. Are you taking any medications for Depression or Anxiety? Do you have any other psychological or psychiatric problems?
There is a strong correlation between Depression, Anxiety, other mental health diagnoses, and sleep problems. It is really important to talk about it. To complicate matters, the medications used to treat these problems may also impact sleep. (See Chapter 17, Medications and Sleep.) If you need drugs for mental health, the benefits of emotional stability and clear thinking generally outweigh the risk of having sleep problems. (See Chapter 15, Psychiatric Problems and Sleep.) It is a delicate balance that should be discussed with your mental healthcare provider and maybe even a sleep specialist.

6. Do you snore? Does your bed partner see you struggling to breathe at night?
Before considering a diagnosis of Insomnia, you may need a sleep study if there is concern about Sleep Apnea.

7. Do you travel across time zones? Have you been on vacation lately?
Jet lag, particularly for people who do it all the time for work, can wreak havoc on the internal clock and sleep

19

timing/coordination. There are techniques to minimize the impact of cross time zone travel. Talking about your travel schedule and how you compensate for sleep is important. (See Chapter 7, Circadian Rhythm Disorders.)

8. Is your preferred time for sleep different from everyone else?
   Circadian rhythm issues (which will be delved into in detail in the Chapter 7 entitled, imaginatively, Circadian Rhythm Disorders) can prevent you from conforming to the "normal" sleep patterns that society and most of us follow. There may not actually be a problem with your sleep, other than having your internal clock set at a different time from everyone else. You just can't sleep when it is "normal" for the rest of the world. Your ability to function suffers because the 8-5 work schedule conflicts with your personal "nighttime." You may need to adjust your work and personal life to synchronize better with your body's internal clock or vice versa.

9. Do you walk, talk, eat, or do anything else in your sleep?
   Being active while you are asleep is clearly contrary to a peaceful night. (These are more fully discussed in Section 5, Odd Sleep Behaviors.)

10. Do you have Narcolepsy symptoms?
    If you are having sleep hallucinations, sleep paralysis, severe daytime sleepiness, and/or physical weakness associated with extremes of emotion, we need to be suspicious of Narcolepsy (see Chapter 13.)

11. Do you have creepy crawly feelings in your legs? Does you bed partner say you move around a lot when sleeping?
    Restless legs are miserable and can keep you awake just when you want to bed down. Repeated movements of the arms or legs during the night disrupt restful sleep. (For info go to Chapter 9, The Movement Parasomnias.)

20

Assuming the questions above don't lead to another diagnosis, we can start to try to figure why you aren't sleeping well.

Q. Who is most likely to have Insomnia?

Anyone, at any age, can suffer from Insomnia. However, Insomnia is more common in people with these characteristics: female gender, middle age or older, Depression, physical inactivity, health problems, social/physical/psychological stress, use of sleep medication, and frequent urination at night. **(Sateia)** That said, there are plenty of women over 50 years of age with medical problems who go to the bathroom frequently at night, worry about their kids, don't work out, and feel like they sleep just fine.

Insomnia can happen to anyone.

Q. My doctor wants me to fill out an Epworth Sleepiness Scale. What is it?

It is the most commonly used screening sleep questionnaire. It is a simple and straightforward way for you to describe how sleepy you feel in very specific situations. You will find it on the next page. Take it if you want.

EPWORTH SLEEPINESS SCALE

How likely are you to doze off or fall asleep in the following situations, in contrast to feeling just tired? This refers to your usual way of life in recent times. Even if you have not done some of these things recently try to work out how they would have affected you. Use the following scale to choose the most appropriate number for each situation:

0 = no chance of dozing
1 = slight chance of dozing
2 = moderate chance of dozing
3 = high chance of dozing

SITUATION	CHANCE OF DOZING
Sitting and reading	_____
Watching TV	_____
Sitting inactive in a public place (e.g. a theater or a meeting)	_____
As a passenger in a car for an hour without a break	_____
Lying down to rest in the afternoon when circumstances permit	_____
Sitting and talking to someone	_____
Sitting quietly after lunch without alcohol	_____
In a car, while stopped for a few minutes in traffic	_____

TOTAL (Greater than 10 = excessive sleepiness)   _____

An elevated Epworth score indicates daytime drowsiness that intrudes on your ability to function and be safe. A diagnosis of Insomnia requires at least some daytime sleepiness that impacts your daily life.

Q. My doctor gave me a form to fill out to record when I am asleep. How do I do that when I am sleeping?

Yes, we sleep doctors like to give our patients lots of homework. But it helps us put together an accurate picture of your sleep.

One of my favorite tools for Insomnia is the Sleep Log or Sleep Diary, pictured on the next page.

We don't expect you to write anything down while you are asleep. For 2 weeks, mark on the graph every time you get into bed, go to sleep, wake up and go back to sleep, and get out of bed. Make your best guess about the times. That includes waking in the middle of the night to go to the bathroom, naps during the day, and nighttime bed, sleep, and wake up times.

The Sleep Log shows the total number of hours of sleep and demonstrates patterns that may lead to a diagnosis. It can also show that you are sleeping better than you think you are, which is helpful in its own way.

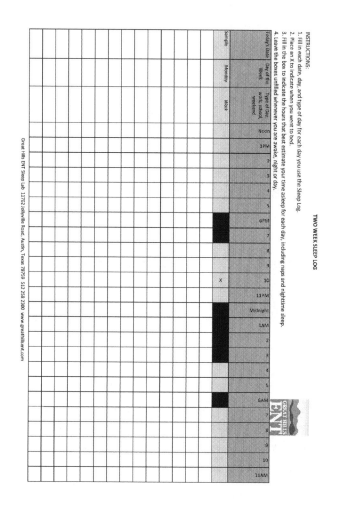

Q. Isn't there an App for that?

Of course there is. In fact there are bunches of them. A quick search of "sleep tracker" at the App Store on my iPhone® pulls up over 200 results.

There are two main kinds of Apps: 1.) Sleep Inducers (e.g.

24

white noise, a calming voice telling you to go to sleep, nature sounds, etc.) and 2.) Sleep Calculators (that tally up the quantity and quality of your sleep.) Many claim they can even follow your sleep stages to determine how deeply you are sleeping.

Those that "measure" sleeping use using some fairly simple software that senses movement called Actigraphy. You may recall the 4 sleep stages in scintillating Chapter 1,"What is Sleep." The deeper you are asleep (moving from Stage 1 to Stage 3) the less you move. In REM (or dream) sleep there should be no activity at all. So if you have a movement sensor on your phone, or on your wrist that is synced with your phone, you can get a general sense of the sleep stages.

The information is interesting to review. It is also nice to compare an app to a sleep log. Any and all information is appreciated and helpful if it gets you a better night's sleep.

Q. **What sort of sleep problems is the doctor likely to see on the Sleep Log?**

The Sleep Log records how much you sleep and when. The patterns that emerge on the graph demonstrate sleep efficiency, or what percentage of your time in bed you are actually asleep. Insomnia is by definition a very inefficient night of sleep.

Everyone's sleep is unique. No two patients come to the doctor with exactly the same sleep problem. But the timing of your sleep disruption helps define if you qualify for one of several categories under the heading of Insomnia. Your sleep pattern provides guidance toward a sleep solution.

Here are some of the most common Insomnia patterns seen on the Sleep Log:

1. **Sleep Onset Insomnia** - difficulty falling asleep at the beginning of the night. (Often associated with anxiety.)
2. **Sleep Maintenance Insomnia** - frequent awakenings throughout the night.
3. **Short Sleep Period** - early morning awakenings with difficulty returning to sleep. (More common in the elderly or depressed people.)

4. **Non-restorative Sleep** - despite adequate sleep quantity recorded on the Sleep Log you feel inadequate quality of sleep. (This occurs for unknown reasons in the absence of any other sleep or medical problem.)
5. **Inadequate Sleep Hygiene** - not going to bed with enough time to sleep before you are supposed to get up. This doesn't count as true Insomnia. If you don't settle down for sleep or plan on enough time in bed to be adequately rested it is your own fault! (See Chapter 2, Advice for Smarter Sleep, and the section about Sleep Hygiene starting on page 11, for a more complete discussion.)

Insomnia Diagnoses

Another way to describe Insomnia is to use the common "official" diagnoses. They are categorized according to the reason for sleep disruption.

Adjustment (Acute) Insomnia –a relatively sudden problem with sleep that occurs because of stressful life situations. Typically, there is a specific event (e.g. divorce, death in the family, job change, move, interpersonal or work strife) that initiates the sleeping difficulty. Stress intrudes on the ability to wind down and relax at bedtime. It is sometimes necessary to seek a doctor's help for a good night's sleep until life returns to normal. This is the most common type of Insomnia and a frequent reason for a short-term prescription of sedative medications. When the stress and life problems resolve, so should the sleep trouble and the need for a drug.

Psychophysiologic Insomnia – a vicious cycle of sleeping difficulty that generates anxiety about being able to fall or stay asleep that in turn disrupts sleep. It is the most distressing form of Insomnia. Psychophsyiologic Insomnia is the persistent and chronic form of Adjustment (Acute) Insomnia.

The process goes like this. Sleep loss seriously impacts daytime function. Nighttime rolls around and you begin to worry that you may again not be able to sleep, so you start to have sleep anxiety. The anxiety keeps you from relaxing and falling asleep. Knowing that your night is once again shot makes you even more anxious. Another poor night of sleep leads to even more daytime problems that make you worry about getting to sleep the next night. This repeating cycle continually disrupts sleep and continually produces anxiety about sleep.

Medication is usually not the best answer for most people with Psychophysiologic Insomnia, though it can have a role in helping to break the cycle. Counseling, about anxiety and worry, and guidance about Sleep Hygiene are the most effective answers.

Idiopathic (A.K.A. we can't figure it out but you really do have Insomnia) **Insomnia** – for unknown reasons, sleep just doesn't happen. No other sleep problems. No worry or anxiety. No recent life stressors. No medical issue or medication to blame. This is often a lifelong sleep problem and medication is usually needed.

Paradoxical Insomnia or **Sleep State Misperception** – the perception that sleep is inadequate when in fact, there are plenty of hours of slumber. This occurs mostly in young and middle aged adults. The Epworth Sleepiness Scale score is high, indicating daytime sleepiness, but the Sleep Log is normal. This one is a bit difficult to explain. Counseling is usually the answer.

Fatal Familial Insomnia – a rare and deadly diagnosis (which means you probably don't have it!) Researchers believe that a prion (sort of a mini virus similar to what causes Mad Cow Disease) is passed down generation to generation, as the name implies. The result of the infection is disruption of normal sleep patterns, nervous system abnormalities, unusual behavior during dreams, and often an inability to sleep at all. Death comes suddenly when fully awake, or during a coma. Nope, you don't want this disease. **(Qi)**

The good news - there have been fewer than 100 cases ever reported in the medical literature. If no one in your family has ever died of this disease (and believe me, you would have heard about it over Thanksgiving dinner), you really don't have to worry.

Q. Why do I have Insomnia?

Good question. You may have one of the diagnoses discussed above, a Primary Insomnia that is a stand-alone problem. Or, your Insomnia may be caused by something else. When you have trouble sleeping because of a medication, a health problem, or a psychiatric illness we call it Secondary Insomnia. We will discuss sleep disruption due to Medical (Chapter 14) and Psychiatric (Chapter 15) problems and Medications (Chapter 17) later in the book.

Q. So how do you treat my Insomnia?

First and foremost, we make sure that you have no other sleep disorder. If your consultation with a sleep doctor does not reveal a diagnosis, you may end up getting a sleep study. It is true that a person who can't sleep is not a great candidate for a <u>sleep</u> study. But if you snore, are overweight, have unexplained and hard to control high blood pressure, new onset heart disease, or have unusual sleeping behaviors (e.g. walking, talking, acting out, or repetitive motions) it might be worthwhile looking in to. If you have another sleep problem, we treat that first. We also make sure that this isn't Secondary Insomnia due to another health problem. If we can't find another reason for your Insomnia, we can start to focus on getting you better.

<u>Insomnia Treatments</u>

"I'm for anything that gets you through the night, be it prayer, tranquilizers, or a bottle of Jack Daniels." Frank Sinatra.

28

1. **Cognitive Behavioral Therapy (CBT)** – (A.K.A. "Helping You Come Up With Better Answers Than Your Current Strategies For Sleep - Therapy.") This is our most effective approach to help you work through your Insomnia. It includes exploring your attitudes toward, and your understanding of, sleep and relaxation – in other words Sleep Hygiene.

    A. **Counseling** - It is important to recognize your mental blocks to sleep. Then you can see that these are the problems, not you. What are your beliefs and attitudes about sleep? How much sleep do you think you need? Why do you feel you are having trouble? Are you afraid of not sleeping? Do you worry about the consequences of being tired during the day? Is this an emotional issue for you?

        What do you do when you can't sleep? Do you get angry? Do you lie in bed with your mind racing? Do you get up to eat or go to the bathroom? Do you take medications or drink alcohol if you can't sleep? Do you check your email or watch TV?

        Exploring these questions and critically discussing them identifies flaws in your sleep logic. Once you see the impact they are having, you are empowered to make necessary changes.

    B. **Relaxation Therapy** – If you have ever taken a yoga class, you will understand this tactic. Unwinding physically helps quiet the mind.

        Progressive relaxation is a nice technique. It goes like this. Get into a comfortable position that you are likely to be in when you fall asleep. Starting at the top of the body and working downward, in sequence, you slowly tighten and then fully release your muscles. First your face, then neck, then hands and arms, chest and back, legs and feet. After this exercise you should feel like a limp rag. Hopefully your mind can take the hint and calm down too.

        Meditation is also included in this category. Inward reflection and contemplation can be very relaxing, preparing you to relax for bedtime. Meditation provides for a state of mental quiet and reduced stress.

C. **Sleep Hygiene** –Take a look at your bedroom
environment. See Chapter 2, Advice for Smarter Sleep, for a
more complete discussion of Sleep Hygiene. But to review,
when you get into bed it should be for intimacy or sleep.
That is all that needs to happen on the mattress. No work, no
TV, no worry, no anything.

Make sure you go to bed when you are tired. Go to
bed early enough to ensure you have at least 8 hours to sleep.
If you are not ready for sleep, don't try. If you can't fall
asleep quickly and easily, get out of bed and do something
else. Lying there worrying about how you can't sleep doesn't
help. The anxiety created by lying in bed not sleeping keeps
you from sleeping! Don't do that.

BOX: Online Insomnia Therapy.

Self-paced, private, internet-based Cognitive Behavioral
Therapy is now available.

SHUTi uses current research and a scientifically validated
approach to Insomnia treatment. There are 6 one-hour
introductory modules, called Cores, which educate about sleep
and sleep problems. Once those are completed, daily sleep logs
are entered and suggestions are made. Progress is easily followed.
This is a pay site, $135 as of this writing. But if this is an
approach that appeals to you, try it. shuti.me

Another option is cbtforinsomnia.com. Costing only
$34.95, this one was developed at Harvard Medical School. It
replicates the 5 visit treatment plan used in Boston for many
patients successfully.

2. **Sleep Restriction and Stimulus Control** – This therapy is
reserved for extreme situations. A sleep specialist sets up a schedule
that purposefully and significantly limits your sleep to much less
than you should be getting. No daytime naps are allowed. When you
finally make it to bed, if you can't sleep you leave at once and only
return when you can hardly keep your eyes open. The goal is to have

you so tired that you fall asleep when you hit the pillow. Period. Solid, consolidated, uninterrupted sleep results because you are so deprived.

Initially, sleep is limited to only 4 hours a night. It may sound cruel to keep an Insomniac from sleeping, but shear exhaustion the day after a short night makes it easier to fall asleep the next night. Once solid sleep is achieved during that 4 hour period the duration is progressively increased until 7 or 8 hours of uninterrupted sleep happens. You can usually take it from there.

Q. Can't I just take a pill? Seems a lot easier than all of that work!

Sure, you could just take a sleeping pill and go to sleep. But it may not fix your problem. Insomnia is more often than not a problem with your life, or your attitudes about and approaches to sleep. Knocking you out with a pill doesn't get you back on the right track to healthy sleep. And medicated sleep is not normal sleep.

Q. But LOTS of people take sleeping pills. There must be some use for them, isn't there?

Absolutely. In fact we prescribe short-term medications for people who are having severe, Acute Insomnia to get them back to a normal sleep schedule. But this is a short-term fix until you make long-term behavioral changes needed for healthy sleep. If you start a sleeping medication, it is best to stop it as soon as possible.

There certainly is a place for chronic medication for chronic, intractable Insomnia. However, no pills, herbal/over-the-counter/prescription, provide NORMAL sleep. They can knock you out for sure. They don't replace the normal sleep cycles and the restoration of natural, unadulterated sleep.

31

Dr B's Opinion: Sleeping Pills
Sleep medications are among the most frequently prescribed drugs in America. On an annual basis, about 25% of Americans take something to help them sleep. **(Sleep Foundation)**

Is there any harm in taking a sleeping pill? Some media reports might lead you to believe that these pills cause cancer. (CBS News) But, the media doesn't always get it right. There is no credible data to back up this claim.

However, sleeping pills are often not the best long-term solution to Insomnia. Addressing bedtime routines, reducing daily stressors, and treating health problems that get in the way of good sleep is almost always a better answer. Some people do need medication though. And that is OK.

(As an aside, I hope that this information will empower you to better understand your sleep issues. Then you and your doctor can work together to find sleep strategies that work, prescription or not.)

Q. So which pill should my doctor give me if I am having trouble sleeping?

Unfortunately, there is no one-pill-fits-all strategy for helping someone fall or stay asleep. Most of the medications we use for sleep promotion are sedatives. The difference lies in the medication's duration of action.

We try to tailor the sedative effect to the specific need. For instance if you just have trouble falling asleep, very short acting medications (Sonata® (zaleplon) ~ 1 hour, Ambien® (zolpidem) ~ 2 hours, and Halcion® (triazolam) ~ 1.5-5 hours) may be all you need. These help you get to sleep but are quickly out of your system so there usually is no morning hangover.

If you fall asleep but have trouble staying there, we might need to go with something that stays in your system longer. Commonly prescribed medications in this group include Lunesta® (eszipiclone − 5-7 hours), Restoril® (temazepam - 8-20 hours), extended release Ambien CR® (zolpidem - 2.8 hours) and Oleptro® (trazadone - 3-14 hours).

There is even a pill you dissolve under your tongue for middle of the night awakening, Intermezzo® (zolpidem tartrate - 2.5 hours). It is quick to start working and quickly out of your system.

Silenor® (doxepin) is an antidepressant that has found benefit particularly for elderly insomniacs. Low doses improved sleep with no hangover effect. **(Krystal)**

A brand new approach to sleep is now available also. Instead of sedating you, this medication turns off wakefulness. While this may seem a trifling disparity, there is huge difference. Belsomra® (suvorexant) is the first medication of its kind approved in the US for insomnia. It inhibits the action of orexin, a brain chemical that stimulates wakefulness. **(Bennett)** Belsomra® (suvorexant shows a beneficial effect during sleep studies in healthy people. And there are very few side effects at correct doses. (**Sun**)

Talk to your doctor about what you might need based on your sleep pattern. If drug one isn't working for you another might. Make sure you have explored all non-pharmaceutical options before you commit to a medication.

We have a more technical discussion of these medications and their impact on sleep in Chapter 17, Medications and Sleep.

Dr. B: What I Say to Insomniacs

Some of the most miserable patients I see in my practice just can't get to sleep. They are tired, sad, anxious, despondent, and desperate. I have seen tears more than once. They have often lost hope. But medicine is a team sport. If I can get them to work with me, together we can usually make a difference.

Most Insomniacs describe their sleep similarly. Difficulty getting to or staying asleep leads to frustration and anger and anxiety and hopelessness. They really are that torn up by the time they get to me. All of their fixes have thus far failed, or they wouldn't be in my office in the first place.

We go through the usual litany of questions to make sure we aren't missing other problems, like Sleep Apnea, pain, Restless Legs, Narcolepsy, etc. Usually, in the absence of another sleep problem the bottom line is the same. Struggle begets struggle.

Sleeplessness compounds sleeplessness. And the cycle needs to be disrupted.

Hope is a powerful tool in medicine. But, not empty hope. The offer of solutions and reassurance goes a LONG way. Giving reassurance that it will get better is about half of my job. The other half is pointing out flaws in bedtime logic and providing tools to overcome them.

The most important thing for an Insomniac to do is to take emotion out of the situation. It does no good to lie in bed at night, angry with yourself and the world because you can't sleep, which is easier said than done. Bad sleep habits are often long term problems with deeply ingrained patterns of sleep loss and the emotional reaction to it. A night normal of sleep is the goal. The starting point is to keep you from making it worse.

So what to do when you can't sleep? Don't panic. There is a great term to describe the turmoil that accompanies this feeling: "catastrophication." This perfectly portrays the mental chaos an Insomniac experiences at the depths of despair of yet another lost night.

If you are not falling asleep easily, get out of bed and go somewhere else. Do NOT turn on a light to read. Do NOT open a laptop or the refrigerator. (That light exposure stimulates wakefulness.) Go into the living room or another quiet safe place. Sit in the dark and take a few deep breaths. Relax. Breath slowly. And let go of the anger and worry. When you are in a better state of mind, try again. You are in charge of the night. You can make the change. Do not let the frustration and angst of Insomnia win.

Also accept that fixing your Insomnia will take some time. You have been doing this for a long time. If tonight is not the night it all comes together, so be it. One night is not the end of the world. It may seem so at the time, but you have many more to get it right. So write off tonight and start again tomorrow. We will get you there.

Smart Sleep Hygiene is the best fix for your Insomnia. Having a smart and relaxing approach to bedtime is the ultimate answer. Preparing to sleep in the right environment, both mentally and physically, is critical.

Part of your solution may be a sleeping pill. Hopefully, a prescription is a short-term necessity. But if a drug is required for

34

the long term, so what! There is no shame in taking a medication to help with sleep. The alternative is much worse.

Section 3: Snoring and Apnea

"Life is what you make it: If you snooze, you lose; and if you snore, you lose more."
Phyllis George

Chapter 4: Snoring

"Laugh and the world laughs with you, snore and you sleep alone."
Anthony Burgess

Snoring…can be funny, sort of, unless you are keeping your bed partner awake at night. Medically, snoring is probably not a threat to your health. It is a THEM problem, not a YOU problem - except for an exasperated loved one's plans for revenge. The following information is presented to you, the Snorer, in an effort to salvage domestic happiness.

Q. Why do I snore?

Snoring comes from your throat and upper airway. It works like this. During sleep your entire body relaxes, including the back of your tongue and your soft palate (where that hangy-downy-punching-bag thing – the uvula – lives at the back of the throat). When you inhale your throat tissues rattle around to create the racket.

Nasal congestion can take snoring to a whole other level. A blocked nose requires more effort to pull air through it into the lungs. The greater the effort the more the throat collapses. (Try it yourself. Pinch you nose shut and try to inhale. Your palate and tongue are pulled back into the throat.)

Your sleeping position has an influence too. When you lie on your back all of those floppy tissues tend to fall backward, making it even worse.

So to answer your question, you snore because your throat collapses and vibrates while you sleep.

Q. Does my weight have anything to do with my snoring?

It is true that heaviness is correlated with snoring. When you gain weight the fat doesn't just go to your waistline and your thighs. Even neck and throat fat expands further crowding the back of the throat and increasing the volume of your snoring. So if you didn't snore 40 pounds ago, it may be that you won't snore minus 40 pounds from now.

Q. If snoring isn't dangerous, do I have to do anything about it?

Not really, unless it is a threat to domestic bliss and the sleep of your bed partner. In that case, maybe you should. Couples often end up on either end of the house so that both can get some sleep, which is not really conducive to marital happiness. Unfortunately most insurance companies don't cover "spousal discontent" as a medical condition. Because most snoring therapies are expensive and require payment out of pocket, many partners just suffer.

Q. Is there anything that can be done to stop snoring without going to the doctor? Those co-pays are killers.

There are many snoring therapies. Just read the inflight magazine on your next trip. Ads for snoring devices, throat sprays, and snoring clinics are everywhere. Clearly there is a market in the traveling public for anti-snoring remedies. I have an entire chapter dedicated to charlatanism (see Chapter 19: Crazy Quackery and Sleep), much of which is dedicated to sham snoring therapies

I can tell you right now, categorically and without a shade of doubt, there is no effective anti-snore wrist device, nasal clamp, throat spray or other snake oil. They are all bogus.

Q. What kind of doctor helps someone with snoring?

Ask your primary care doctor for a referral to a reputable Ear, Nose, and Throat (ENT) specialist with an interest in snoring and sleep issues. It is helpful to have the one who is suffering (not you, the one who can't sleep because of you) go to the visit also. Since you are not awake when you snore, having someone there to describe the noise is helpful. The ENT will ask bunch of questions about your sleep. Are you sleeping well? Do you awaken refreshed? Do you snore louder when sleeping on your back? Does your bed partner hear you stop breathing? Do you have nasal congestion/allergies/sinus problems? An Epworth Sleepiness Scale (see Chapter 3: Insomnia, to see the questionnaire) may be completed to measure your perception of how sleepy you feel during the day.

Having your bed partner with you plays a vital role in this visit. If he or she is worried that you stop breathing while snoring the possibility of Sleep Apnea is explored. A complete head and neck exam usually follows.

Q. So what are my options, doc?

It depends on what the ENT finds. There are surgical and non-surgical approaches to snoring therapies. Let's start with the ones that don't hurt first.

Non-Operative Treatments for Snoring

Several devices are available that are attractive options: they may actually work, are not invasive, don't require anesthesia, and are relatively inexpensive. No harm in looking into one of these approaches before committing to a procedure.

NASAL MEDICATION FOR ALLERGIES:
Nasal congestion due to allergies or inflammation can cause or exacerbate snoring. Millions of people suffer from seasonal and perennial allergies. Millions more have nasal inflammation from smog, fumes, and other environmental irritants.

Allergy treatment with a nasal medication is a good start. If a safe, topical nasal antihistamine (like Astelin®/Astepro® (azleastine), or Patanase® (olopatadine)) or steroid (Q'Nasl® (beclomethasone), Nasonex® (mometasone), Nasacort AQ® (triamcinolone), or Flonase® (fluticasone)) or combination (like Dymista® (fluticasone + azelastine)) do the trick, you don't need surgery. If medication fails and you do have a physical airway blockage, surgery is an option.

NASAL DILATOR STRIPS:
Athletes frequently use these to improve nasal airflow. And for that purpose these strips are very effective. **(Wong)** Breathe Right Strips® are the most popular brand advertised. There are some studies, funded by the manufacturer, that claim that these dramatically improve snoring. I am always skeptical of industry-funded research. Anecdotally, my patients say they work. Worth a try.

PROVENT® and THERAVENT®:

   These are relatively new and novel approaches to snoring treatment. Provent® is marketed for snoring relief and as an alternative to CPAP for Sleep Apnea. Theravent® is used only for snoring. Both devices consist of single use patches that fit on the nostrils (Provent®) or over the end of the nose (Theravent®) to act as a one-way airflow valve. You inhale as you normally do through the patch on the nose. When you exhale the valve closes and air is diverted through the mouth. Initially, as you are trying to exhale, air pressure inflates your throat. Eventually, the mouth opens up and you exhale. That dilation of the throat prevents collapse and quiets the noise.

   One good study showed some success treating both snoring and very mild Sleep Apnea with Provent®. It did not cure Apnea or eliminate oxygen problems with OSA but there was improvement. The amount of time spent snoring was really reduced, though. **(Rosenthal)** It is also very safe and easy to use.

   These devices take some getting used to. Provent® sends you a starter set that slowly increases the resistance on exhalation. This helps you ease into sleeping with them on. Theravent® has different "strengths," Lite, Regular, and Max, depending on your need.

PROVENT®   THERAVENT®

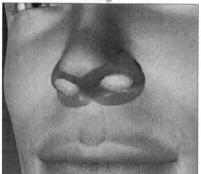
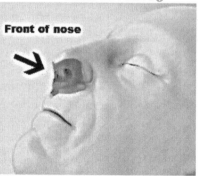

(used with permission from Provent Therapy, Inc. proventtherapy.com)

(used with permission from Theravent, Inc. theravent.com)

   The Provent® system is prescribed by a physician. Theravent® is over the counter. Neither are usually covered by insurance plans.

The upside of these devices is that they are removable and don't require a procedure of any sort. But, they can be costly over the long haul. Remember, though, we are preserving your relationship. Your partner is worth it.

TONGUE RETAINER:
One of my favorites is a suction cup device, the aveo TSD®. It grabs the tip of the tongue and pulls it out of the mouth. When the tongue is pulled forward it can't collapse into the throat to make noise. I agree, it doesn't sound very comfortable. But it works well if you are willing to wear it. A doctor's prescription is required. So you need to see someone who is familiar with the device, like a Sleep Medicine specialist.

One study looking at the use of this device for Obstructive Sleep Apnea demonstrated improvement in snoring loudness. It also showed improvement in Sleep Apnea, **(Lazard)** but not enough to consider this as a stand alone treatment. For what it is worth, my patients who use the aveoTSD® for snoring have had success, as measured by their spouse's happiness. The only downsides are possible temporary irritation under the tongue, dry mouth, and drooling.

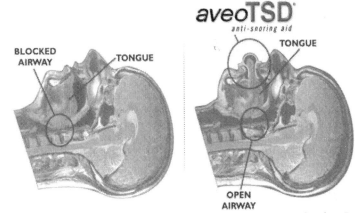

(Used with permission Innovative Health /technologies Ltd)

MANDIBULAR ADVANCEMENT DEVICE (MAD):
There are several oral/dental devices that are available on the Internet (most likely not going to work) or from a dentist who

41

specializes in this sort of thing (much more likely to work). An upper and lower mouthpiece fitted to your teeth is connected to a screw crank. The lower jaw is progressively pulled forward with the crank. This action draws the tongue and its connections to the palate up and out of the throat – snoring improved! And they do work if you can wear them. An analysis of the research showed a 45% reduction in snoring, on average. **(Hoffstein)**

Drawbacks for the MAD are few, but occasionally daunting. Jaw joint (TMJ) pain, tooth pain, bite misalignment (due to the pulling forces on the teeth), dry mouth, and drooling are possible. **(Doff)** Fortunately, these problems are rare.

If you are interested in this approach, I advise you to find a dentist with the special expertise needed to fit you correctly. Being under the care of an expert diminishes the likelihood of a problem with your jaw and teeth.

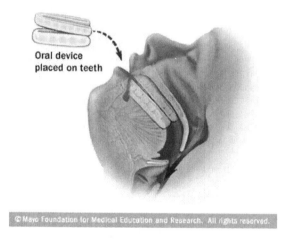

Oral device placed on teeth

(Used with permission from "Obstructive sleep apnea." http://www.mayoclinic.org/diseases-conditions/obstructive-sleep-apnea/multimedia/oral-device/img-20007681)

Surgical Treatments for Snoring

There are several surgical approaches to snoring. They are often effective and occasionally really painful. And remember, they are probably not going to be covered by insurance.

Working from the top down...

NOSE:

It is rare that the nose cause snoring all by itself. But, nasal blockage does make snoring significantly worse. When the nose is blocked it is harder to inhale which makes the throat collapse more. Nasal congestion arises from anatomy problems (for example a deviated septum or enlarged turbinates, see below) or some sort of inflammation (like allergies or sinus infections - see non-surgical snoring therapies above). If there are no adequate medical answers, surgical improvement of the nasal airway can make a difference.

> **Septoplasty with Turbinate Reduction**. Straightening a crooked septum and reducing turbinates improves the nasal airspace and therefore breathing.
>
> **Anesthesia:** General.
>
> **Setting:** Operating Room, outpatient.
>
> **Recovery:** 7-10 days.
>
> **Pain Level:** 5/10. Pain meds for 3-5 days.
>
> **Risks:** Bleeding (extremely rare), Infection (extremely rare), continued nasal obstruction (rare).
>
> **Effectiveness:** Patient satisfaction with this procedure is very high. ~50% reduction in bed partner reported snoring in patients with sleep apnea who had nasal airway surgery. Not too many scientific studies are available. **(Rappai)** However, nasal airway surgery seems to be associated with better sleep quality and restfulness. **(Stapleton)**

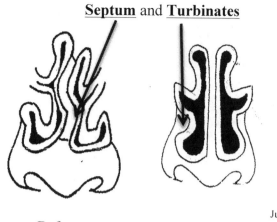

Septum and **Turbinates**

Julia Argent

Before   After

THROAT: Large, floppy palatal tissues and tonsils are prime offenders when talking about snoring. Treatment of these areas is not for the faint of heart...

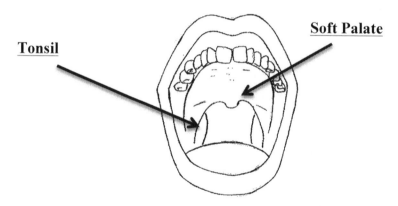

Tonsil   **Soft Palate**

Tonsils: Located at the back of the throat on the sides. If they are big they block the airway.

> **Tonsillectomy.** Removing large tonsils from the throat opens it and decreases snoring.
> **Anesthesia:** General.
> **Setting:** Operating Room, outpatient.
> **Recovery:** 10-14 days.

Pain Level: 9-10/10. Pain meds for 10-14 days. Yes, this is a very painful procedure. Missing work for 2 weeks is not unheard of. You really have to commit to having this one done.

Risks: Bleeding (1%), continued snoring (very unlikely.)

Effectiveness: There is little data on adult snoring therapy with tonsillectomy alone. Experience supports this procedure if there is massive enlargement and no evidence of sleep apnea.

Before   After

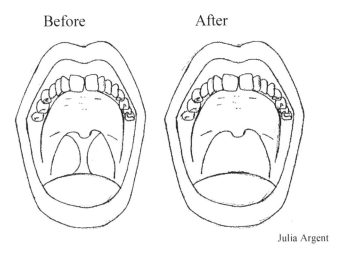

Julia Argent

Palate: A big, floppy, soft palate is the most common cause of snoring. Reducing and stiffening that extra tissue decreases the noise. A smaller and firmer palate is a quieter palate. There are a variety of options to improve this area, some more invasive than others. Common to all of these procedures is an injury to the palatal tissue. With injury comes scarring. Scars tend to shrink and stiffen as they heal. This makes for less vibration and noise. All of these are office procedures done under local anesthesia.

<u>**Laser Assisted Uvulopalatopharyngoplasty (LAUP).**</u> A laser is used to scar and decrease the amount of palate soft tissue.

Anesthesia: Local.

Setting: Office, outpatient.

Recovery: 10-14 days.

Pain Level: 8/10. Pain meds for up to a week.

Risks: Bleeding (<1%), continued snoring, airway fire due to laser (extremely unlikely), nasal regurgitation with swallowing (extremely unlikely). (Few doctors are still performing LAUPs because of cost and safety.)
Effectiveness: ~50% decrease in snoring. **(Macdonald)**

Before   After

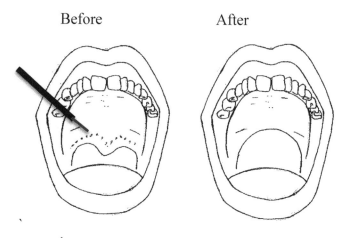

Julia Argent

Palatal Pillars. Many of the "snore clinics" that advertise specialize in this technique. The palatal pillar procedure is reasonably effective and has relatively little overall risk. It is often very expensive.

Small tunnels are created in the soft palate, into which 3 small pieces of braided polyester (recycled from old leisure suits?) are inserted. An intense scarring reaction causes stiffening of the palate.

Anesthesia: Local.
Setting: Office, outpatient.
Recovery: 10-14 days.
Pain Level: 2-4/10. Pain meds for a few days occasionally.
Risks: Bleeding (extremely unlikely), continued snoring, rejection of pillar material (~4%)
Effectiveness: About 50% long term reduction in snoring volume. **(Stale)**

Before   After

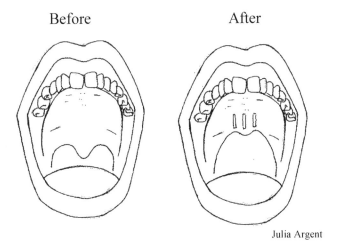

Julia Argent

Radiofrequency Palate Ablation. A probe is inserted into the soft palate. Radiofrequency energy is used to injure, scar, and stiffen the tissues. This makes the palate more rigid and resistant to vibration and snoring.

Anesthesia: Local.

Setting: Office, outpatient.

Recovery: 10-14 days.

Pain Level: 5-7/10. Pain meds for up to a week on occasion.

Risks: Bleeding (extremely unlikely), continued snoring (50-75% success rate)

Effectiveness: 42% with complete snoring resolution, 52% with reduced snoring. **(Carroll)**

47

Before　　　　　　　After

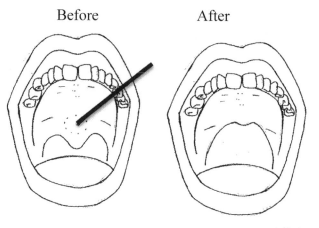

Julia Argent

Injection Snoreplasty. This technique injects either pure
　　　alcohol or Sotradecol® (sodium tetradecyl sulfate) as
　　　a scarring agent into the palatal tissues. The injury
　　　shortens and stiffens the palate. Up to 3 injections
　　　may be needed for the effect.
Anesthesia: Local.
Setting: Office, outpatient.
Recovery: 7 days.
Pain Level: 5-7/10. Pain meds for up to a week on occasion.
Risks: Bleeding (extremely unlikely), continued snoring
Effectiveness: Decreased snoring in ~90% initially and
　　　~75% long term. **(Brietzke)**

Before　　　　　　　After

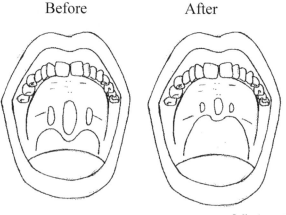

Julia Argent

Bottom Line:

   All of these techniques work for snoring. As you can, see all have a failure rate. They are relatively safe and simple. They are also expensive and insurance does not pay for them. But there are times when extreme measures are needed to insure domestic bliss.

To summarize…

Anatomical Site	Non-surgical	Surgical
Nose	Nasal allergy control – Medications to reduce inflammation and improve airflow. Nasal dilator strips – Opening the nasal airway physically to improve nasal airflow. Provent®- Positive pressure to keep the airway open on exhalation .	Septoplasty with turbinate reduction – Anatomical obstruction is removed to improve nasal airflow.
Mouth/Tongue	Aveo TSD® - Pulls the tongue up and out of the throat to prevent collapse. Mandibular Advancement Device (MAD) – Pulls the lower jaw forward, and the tongue and palate along with it, preventing collapse of the airway.	
Throat		Tonsillectomy – Enlarged and obstructive tonsils are removed to open the throat and prevent collapse. Laser Assisted Uvulopalatpplasty (LAUP), Palatal Pillars, Radiofrequency Palate Ablation, Injection Snoreplasy– All of these intend to injury the floppy soft palate to induce stiffening and prevention of collapse and vibration.

Chapter 5: Obstructive Sleep Apnea

"Hark, how hard he fetches breath."
William Shakespeare, *King Henry IV, Part 1*

Obstructive Sleep Apnea: Definition

This is the ugly and dangerous big brother of snoring. Sleep Apnea is a real and often unrecognized problem. Fortunately there is growing public and medical awareness of the diagnosis and the consequences of untreated Sleep Apnea. As we discussed in Chapter 4, snoring is a THEM problem. Obstructive Sleep Apnea (OSA), on the other hand, is a YOU and THEM problem. Read on to see if your life and health are at risk.

Q. Does everybody who snores have sleep apnea?

Snoring is sleep apnea "lite." Like with many things, there is a spectrum of severity. At the quiet end is that cute little sound your wife makes after she falls asleep on the couch. On the other end is real Obstructive Sleep Apnea, which is a big deal.

Snoring < Mild OSA < Moderate OSA < Severe OSA

Q. What is Obstructive Sleep Apnea?

The term "Apnea" is a medical term that breaks down as follows: "A-" means "no" and "-PNEA" refers to "breathing." During an "apnea" the airway is completely collapsed so that there is no airflow. A lesser, but equally disruptive, breathing problem called "hypopnea" also happens in Sleep Apnea. Breaking down this term gives us "HYPO-" or " less" and "-PNEA" referring again to "breathing." These are partial obstructions. Air still moves, but just barely. While not as dramatic as apneas, hypopneas are just as problematic to sleep and health. Every one of these obstruction events, partial or complete, disrupts sleep - forcing you to wake up a little bit to breath again.

Also, if you are not breathing, it follows that you won't be inhaling oxygen and exhaling carbon dioxide. Normally we have quite lot of oxygen in our blood. We refer to this as the oxygen saturation percentage. A healthy person is 98-100% full of oxygen while awake. As breathing is not as deep or frequent during sleep, a healthy person is in the 92-97% range overnight. During apneas and hypopneas, oxygen levels drop, sometimes to dangerous levels.

As you might expect, not breathing, having interrupted sleep, and not getting enough oxygen, over and over again every night, is just not good for you.

Q. Sometimes I wake up feeling like I am choking to death! What keeps me from dying in my sleep when I have an apnea?

As scary as that experience is, your brain insures that you make it through the night. You will take another breath. Your brain's control centers take notice if you aren't breathing. As oxygen levels decrease and carbon dioxide levels rise, alarms start to go off. Your brain leaps into action. "Hey, take a breath!" decreasing your level of sleep to break the obstruction. You rarely fully awaken (though those choking episodes you describe are the exceptions to that rule). Most of the time your sleep is disrupted just enough to return muscle tone to the throat. Then you breathe again…until the next apnea.

This cycle of airway obstruction and sleep disruption makes it difficult to descend into those restful, deeper stages of sleep. Thus, you are really tired after a night of Obstructive Sleep Apnea.

Q. What is Central Sleep Apnea (CSA)?

Central sleep apnea (CSA) occurs when the brain forgets to tell you to breathe. The controls centers are not functioning correctly. It is very rare, seen after brain injuries, some heart conditions, and in unusual syndromes. We will address these conditions and their consequences in Chapter 6, Central Sleep Apnea.

Q. It seems like everybody I talk to these days has Sleep Apnea. Is it really that common?

Yes. A survey of thousands of adults taken in 2006 found that 4.7% of Americans had already been diagnosed with Sleep Apnea: 14,000,000 people! **(Punjabi)** This means that about 1 in 20 Americans have the diagnosis. And, that probably underestimates the number of people truly affected.

Q. My husband snores so loudly I have moved out of our bedroom. Help! Does this mean he has Sleep Apnea?

If his noise is awakening the neighbors you should be suspicious. Sleep technicians grade snoring during studies on a 4-point scale. Level 1 snoring is quiet, fairly rare, and not disruptive. Level 4 is the snoring equivalent of a jet engine. You are more likely to have Sleep Apnea if you snore at DEFCON 4 (describe as "heroic" snoring - not sure why these people are heroes – go figure). But at the other extreme, quiet snoring does not exclude the possibility of Sleep Apnea.

Q. What are the risk factors for developing Sleep Apnea?

WEIGHT:
The more a person weighs the more likely they have Sleep Apnea. But it is more than just weight. The BMI (body mass index) is a more accurate indicator of risk. While this measurement is not perfect, the BMI tries to make sense of your weight in the context of your height. The BMI formula is weight divided by the squared measurement of height. It is a good and convenient measurement of body fat.

$$BMI = \frac{Weight}{Height^2}$$

According to the Centers for Disease Control (CDC) BMI ranges are categorized as follows:

BMI	Weight Status
Below 18.5	Underweight
18.5 – 24.9	Normal
25.0 – 29.9	Overweight
30.0 and Above	Obese

Take BMI with a grain of salt though. Famously, in his playing days, Michael Jordan was overweight according to this classification. His BMI was 25 due to his height (6' 6") and weight (216 lbs.). But, he was almost pure muscle. Many athletes have elevated BMIs because of their muscle mass, which is much greater than most of us armchair quarterbacks. But, most of the people who are overweight and snoring are not Michael Jordan. So we take these numbers in the context of the whole patient. Anyone who treats sleep disorders can cite examples of the obese man who sleeps quietly and soundly and the skinny woman who snores like a freight train.

That said, the BMI is a generally useful and easy measure of body fat and an elevated number is strongly associated with OSA.

NECK CIRCUMFERENCE:

Men with shirt sizes 18" or higher are at increased risk. That may explain why there is a surprisingly high rate of OSA in professional football players. Don't be shocked if your neck is measured when you go in for your visit with the sleep doctor.

AGE AND GENDER:

Men are significantly more likely to have sleep apnea. It may have to do with how male weight and fat are distributed. Or men may have different throat structures. Regardless, men are more commonly affected, especially in middle age. Sleep apnea occurs in any decade and gender, but men in their 50s are the most typical group.

ANATOMY:
Some people just have the wrong mouth and throat anatomy for sleep. For example: a short jaw does not support the tongue in a forward position. As the tongue falls back it obstructs the throat. Or there are huge tonsils, or lots of extra palatal tissues. Or all of the above may come together to create the obstructions. There are no accurate ways to measure how much one part causes Apnea versus another. But it is usually pretty easy to see by the trained eye of a Sleep Specialist.

NASAL OBSTRUCTION:
Finally, nasal congestion also contributes. Go ahead and try it. Pinch your nose shut and try to breathe in. If you do this repeatedly you can feel the tongue get pulled back and the throat collapse. Nasal congestion worsens airway collapse in OSA.

Q. My dad had sleep apnea. Will I?

While sleep apnea is usually not part of a defined disease or syndrome, I have lots of patients who find that this is a family affair. If your father's airway is prone to collapse, you anatomy may be similar and do the same. But remember, half your genes come from Mom. Just be observant for the signs and symptoms of Sleep Apnea (see below). If you, or your family is concerned, take it seriously and seek out a professional opinion. As you will see, not treating Sleep Apnea can be a real impact on your health. So if Dad has it, you may as well.

Q. What other clues are there to sleep apnea?

Almost all patients who have real OSA are sleepy, whether or not they admit to it. (Men are particularly good at denial). This is a common office scenario: Husband - denies any problems with snoring, tiredness, or lack of energy; Wife - sits behind him silently nodding yes to all of those questions.

Asking for help is not a masculine thing to do. But no matter how tough a person is, one can't help but be tired if sleep is disrupted 5 or more times per hour at night. Work efficiency and personal relationships suffer. Being focused and alert is a challenge. Caffeine is a common crutch – which helps, but not nearly as much as a good night's sleep.

Q. At my doctor's office I had to answer a questionnaire about how sleepy I am. What is that all about?

This scale is useful for any sleep issues. It is a simple and straightforward way for a person to self-describe his or her sleepiness. It is the most commonly used questionnaire in sleep medicine. You can see it, and maybe take the test, on the next page.

EPWORTH SLEEPINESS SCALE

How likely are you to doze off or fall asleep in the following situations, in contrast to feeling just tired? This refers to your usual way of life in recent times. Even if you have not done some of these things recently try to work out how they would have affected you. Use the following scale to choose the most appropriate number for each situation:

0 = no chance of dozing
1 = slight chance of dozing
2 = moderate chance of dozing
3 = high chance of dozing

SITUATION	CHANCE OF DOZING
Sitting and reading	_____
Watching TV	_____
Sitting inactive in a public place (e.g. a theater or a meeting)	_____
As a passenger in a car for an hour without a break	_____
Lying down to rest in the afternoon when circumstances permit	_____
Sitting and talking to someone	_____
Sitting quietly after lunch without alcohol	_____
TOTAL (Greater than 10 = excessive sleepiness.)	_____

People who score over ten are "pathologically sleepy." One word of caution about this little questionnaire; the severity of your sleepiness score is completely up to you. If you are one of those people who minimizes your physical complaints and just works through whatever problem you have (e.g. a man) you tend to score lower. If you are VERY in tune with your body and tend to focus on how you feel you will tend to score higher.

Q. I keep having dreams that I am drowning or that someone is trying to strangle me to death. I am really freaked out and kind of afraid to go to sleep. Is that normal?

Obstructive Apnea is worse during the deepest and most relaxed stage, REM or dream sleep. Incorporating real choking and gasping into your dream is very frightening. Awakening during this struggle intensifies the experience, so much so that some people develop severe anxiety about sleep. It can get so bad that they develop a fear of dying during sleep. The best way to get rid of this problem is to get rid of the Obstructive Sleep Apnea!

Q. My doctor is worried about my sleep because of my blood pressure, why?

High blood pressure and Sleep Apnea go hand in hand. In fact, snoring patients with otherwise unexplained or hard to control blood pressure should have a sleep study. Treating Sleep Apnea helps bring down blood pressure in a person with both problems. (**Marin**) So there is good reason to be suspicious and concerned.

Q. Does sleep apnea <u>cause</u> the elevation of blood pressure?

Yes, and a lot more. Lets look at a single apnea event to illustrate just how the damage is done.

There you are, peacefully minding your own business, snoring, disrupting your bed partner's sleep, and disrupting the neighbor's sleep, when suddenly you have an apnea. Breathing is obstructed so oxygen levels drop and carbon dioxide levels rise. As you try to break the apnea and breathe again, you get stressed, as if you are afraid or under attack. An adrenalin rush occurs as you break the obstruction and take that next breath. The adrenalin causes blood pressure to rise and the heart rate to go up. The heart beats harder in a low oxygen environment against a now higher blood pressure.

Imagine that occurring every night for the rest of your life. Over the long term, repeated assaults on the heart and circulation cause permanent damage. Blood vessel tone increases, maintaining a higher blood pressure day and night. The blood vessels themselves are injured and are prone to clotting. That means that you are at risk for stroke and heart attack. Over the years, that workload on the heart increases the risk of heart failure. You get the picture. The risks are real.

Imagine that sequence of events occurring every 12 minutes while you sleep. This is the <u>mildest</u> form of sleep apnea. That process is repeated 20 or 40 or even 100 or more times per hour in people with more severe Sleep Apnea.

Sleep apnea should not be taken lightly. Diagnosis and treatment can save your life.

Q. What is Pickwickian Syndrome?

This is the most severe form of sleep related breathing problems. It refers to a character named Joe in Charles Dickens novel "The Pickwick Papers." Joe is an obese young man, red in the face, always hungry, and always falling asleep, even while standing. He is teased about his condition in the book. But Joe had a real and often fatal problem. The medical term for this malady is Obesity Hypoventilation (not breathing deeply) Syndrome (OHS). It affects morbidly obese people who weigh so much they cannot breathe effectively awake or asleep. Chronic and persistent low blood oxygen (↓) and high carbon dioxide (↑) blunts the brain control center's drive to breathe. To make matters even worse, excessive weight often leads to severe Obstructive Sleep Apnea. Chronic daytime sleepiness, heart failure, leg swelling, headaches, and depression also occur. If untreated, this is a fatal condition.

Management is multifaceted. CPAP/BiPAP(described later on in this chapter) are the mainstays of therapy. It may be necessary

59

to bypass the obstructed airway with a tracheotomy. Radical measures for weight loss are prescribed, including stomach surgeries and medically controlled diets.

Dickens may have thought it was comical to see a person with what we have now termed Pickwickian Syndrome. We know better.

Q. Is Sleep Apnea dangerous?

See the two answers above. But there even are additional concerns! Daytime sleepiness caused by Sleep Apnea puts you and others at risk on the road. Drowsy driving is a serious problem. Falling asleep behind the wheel is clearly a danger to everyone. **(Howard)** Imagine a bus or truck driver with untreated Apnea.

Fortunately for the traveling public, affected professional drivers often must prove successful treatment of Obstructive Sleep Apnea. Proof of treatment is easy to find. Modern CPAP machines provide data about hours of use and effectiveness. Also, if the driver has a surgery or other non-CPAP therapy, follow up sleep studies are used to determine cure. There is also a specific sleep study, called a Maintenance of Wakefulness Test (MWT) described later, that can further determine treatment effect.

Q. How is obstructive Sleep Apnea related to acid reflux?

Imagine an apnea. Trying desperately to inhale against a collapsed airway sucks your stomach up into your chest. That forceful effort also pulls stomach acid upward. In susceptible people, Sleep Apnea almost guarantees reflux. Successful treatment of OSA often improves acid regurgitation. This is just another benefit to taking care of your Sleep Apnea.

Obstructive Sleep Apnea: Diagnosis

If there is real concern about Obstructive Sleep Apnea, testing is needed. It takes a lot of work, but something as important as your health deserves the effort.

Q. Do I need a sleep study?

Your medical history and examination determine your need for a sleep study. Are you snoring, struggling to breathe, gasping and choking at night, hard to awaken in the morning, grumpy during the day, falling asleep watching TV, and/or depressed? Do you have nasal congestion? Do you still have your tonsils? How is your weight – going up? Do you have new or worsening medical problems? New onset or uncontrolled high blood pressure or severe heart disease?

Your bed partner's input is also really important. Having him or her describe your behavior in sleep is something you can't do. Are you restless? Do you stop breathing? Has your snoring worsened?

All of the answers help describe your sleep (or lack thereof). A general exam, with an emphasis on your nose and throat, reveals areas of potential obstruction. Your doctor considers all of these factors before advising a sleep study.

Q. My doctor is concerned about my sleep and is sending me to a lab for a study. I don't like the idea of going to a "lab" like some rat! What is a sleep lab?

This is an overnight facility that monitors and evaluates your sleep. It can be located in a hospital, a doctor's office, or in a freestanding sleep lab facility. Yes, you need to spend the night there. Yes, it is a little weird going to a place, getting wired up, and being told by a total stranger to go to sleep. However, a good lab does all it can to make the environment safe, calm and as comfortable as possible. You will have a private room, too. You arrive about an hour prior to your usual bedtime to be educated about the study, get wired up, and prepare for sleep.

Q. I am afraid I won't be able to sleep. Should I take something to knock me out?

You should try to avoid taking something if it is not part of your usual sleep routine. Since you don't routinely take a sedative, it may alter your sleep and the information we are looking for. Some labs have a standing order for a sleep medication like Ambien® (zolpidem) or Lunesta® (eszoplicone) in case someone just can't get to sleep.

Sorry, if your nighttime routine normally includes a drink. The sleep technician can't double as a bartender. A sleeping pill may have to suffice.

Most people get reasonable sleep despite the environment and wires. For one thing, you are there because you are chronically sleep deprived. Falling asleep is typically not a problem.

However, some people have the "First Night Effect" and can't sleep. The lab environment and monitoring devices are very different from your normal night. It is a strange experience just to be there. If sleep fails you the first time around, the second night is usually much easier and more successful.

Q. I normally do take a sleeping pill. Should I on the night of the study?

Yes. Take your normal medications, even if that includes something to help you sleep.

Q. What happens during a diagnostic sleep study in a sleep lab?

Diagnostic sleep studies give your doctor a very complete picture of your sleep. A wide array of monitors measure many different aspects of your slumber.

A certified sleep technician is present in the lab all night (though not in your room – don't worry). This person, who is responsible for applying all of the equipment, will be there to educate you and do their best to make the experience as stress free and comfortable as possible. He or she also troubleshoots the many monitors you wear while you are sleeping.

Sleep Study Monitors

Sleep studies are extremely technical undertakings. About twenty different channels of information feed back wirelessly to the lab computer to create a complex and nuanced picture of your entire night of sleep. The standard monitors and how they work are listed below – if you want all the technical details.

Brain Activity

Electroencephalogram (EEG): leads are affixed to your scalp in very specific areas. These sticky little pads detect the electrical activity generated by the brain (waves).

- The information shows how and when your brain enters sleep and defines each of the sleep stages. The amount and distribution of those stages are also recorded.

Breathing

Breathing Effort: recorded from movement-sensing bands positioned around your chest and belly. Normal coordination of breathing is disrupted during an apnea.

Airflow: measured by a tube placed under your nose. During apnea, or hypopnea, there is no, or limited, airflow.

Blood oxygen saturation: documented by a simple probe attached to your earlobe or finger. The monitor gauges the amount of oxygen in your blood.

- Combining breathing effort, oxygen levels, and airflow information defines an obstructive event

Muscle Activity

Electromyography

(EMG): sensors placed over chin and front of the leg measure electrical activity created by muscle activity. They also determine the presence of, and tally the number of, repetitive limb movements.

- Muscle activity helps define sleep stages. There is none in Stage REM. Repetitive limb movements help diagnose treatable sleep disorders.

Eye Movement

Electrooculography (EOG): sensors placed above and below the side of the eyes track the presence and pattern of eye movements during and while entering sleep.

- The eyes are important to defining REM sleep.

Cardiac Activity

Electrocardiogram (EKG): leads are placed on your chest to record and measure heart rate and rhythm.

- Heart rate varies with sleep stages. Heart rhythm disturbances are more common at night and in the presence of Sleep Apnea.

Sleep Position Sensor

Body position has a big influence on snoring and apnea in many people. Being on your back (supine) may exacerbate obstructions.

Q. Will I be able to sleep with all of that stuff on me?

It normally it takes a person 15 to 20 minutes to fall asleep.

People who need a sleep study are usually very tired because of their Sleep Apnea, Narcolepsy, or other sleep disorder. It doesn't matter where they are or even what time it is. If the opportunity comes to get some shut-eye, it will happen in a heartbeat – even with a bunch of wires and monitors attached!

Q. Is it possible to do a home sleep study?

Yes. Insurance companies often prefer these to more complete in lab studies. Why? You guessed it – they're cheaper. But you get what you pay for. On the one hand, a home study is almost like taking a chest X-ray of only one lung. You can't get the whole picture. On the other hand, they are reasonably good at determining the presence or absence of Sleep Apnea. **(Ayappa)** They fall short when looking for other sleep diagnoses though. Most sleep specialists prefer in-lab studies because they gather significantly more information about your sleep.

There are many home sleep study devices available, some better than others. Generally, they have limited data acquisition capacity. As opposed to an in-lab study that assesses about 20 channels of information, most in-home screens usually gather only 4: nasal airflow, oxygen saturation, snoring sound levels, and heart rate.

Others claim to simulate an in lab study, providing much more data. Basically, you go to a real sleep lab, put on their usual monitors, and then go home to sleep.

The advantage of a home sleep study is that being in your own bed should be a more relaxing and comfortable sleeping environment than the lab. And being in your own bed <u>may</u> represent a more usual night of sleep despite the monitors. Getting more than one night of data is easier also.

The disadvantage of a home study, other than limited data acquisition, is that you are alone with a highly technical piece of equipment. If there is a problem during the night <u>you</u> have to deal with it. One device has a feature that wakes you up if it isn't working right and tells you how to fix it. If your study is being followed by a remote sleep tech via the Internet, you may get phone calls to change position or reset a probe. I have had several patients come to me after experiencing one of these studies. They did not

65

have a good night of sleep, despite being in their own bed. The in home study was neither restful nor representative of their sleep.

Q. I had a high resolution oximetry test. Is it the same as a home sleep study?

High res oximetry is a nice screen to look for the oxygen problems you often see with Sleep Apnea. It does not replace an a sleep study, but is a convenient and simple screen to find out if there is concern in the first place. Most likely, if it is abnormal, you will be getting a "real" study (home or otherwise) in the near future.

Q. What does it mean that my Obstructive Sleep Apnea (OSA) is mild/moderate/severe?

Sleep Apnea severity is determined mainly by two metrics: breathing disruptions and oxygen levels.

The Apnea Hypopnea Index (AHI) calculates the number of times your breathing is disrupted. (It is the total number of events divided by the number of hours of sleep during the study). An apnea or hypopnea "incident" is defined very precisely: airflow is obstructed or severely limited for at least 10 seconds, oxygen levels falls by at least 4%, and sleep is disrupted when the event is broken. It is a significant occurrence. The numbers of events (AHI) combined with oxygen saturation levels together determine the level of your Sleep Apnea.

Most Sleepologists (OK, I just made that name up) believe that there must be 5 or more disrupted breathing episodes (obstructed or ineffective breaths associated with oxygen desaturation as defined above) per hour to get a diagnosis of OSA. That may seem like quite a few at first glance. But, the body tolerates less than five without significant medical complications.

The usually accepted sleep apnea severity designations are as follows.

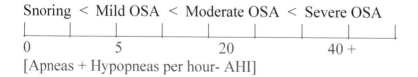

Snoring < Mild OSA < Moderate OSA < Severe OSA

0	5	20	40 +

[Apneas + Hypopneas per hour- AHI]

If there are a relatively small number of apneas but significant decreases in blood oxygen levels we are likely to upgrade the severity designation. Lower oxygen levels put more stress on your cardiovascular system (heart and blood vessels) even if there are not as many breathing events through the night.

Q. The testing is done. I have Sleep Apnea. What's next?

Ideally you sit down with your sleep doctor and discuss the situation. You probably didn't go to medical school. But even if you did, it is helpful having someone interpret the results for you. Better decisions are made when you understand the severity of the problem and your risks going forward. What can you do with your lifestyle and health that might improve your sleep? What are the options for therapy? Where do you go from here? Your doctor should lay it all out for you and help you make smart decisions for your health.

Obstructive Sleep Apnea: Treatment

Now that you have a diagnosis you need to discuss treatment options with your sleep specialist. You may be thinking, "Just fix it, doc!" It is not always that easy.

Broadly, there are non-surgical approaches, like CPAP, dental devices, and positional therapy. And there are surgical options. Occasionally combining more than one treatment works best. There is a trial and error aspect to finding the right therapy or combination that works for you. The severity of your Sleep Apnea also influences your options.

All sleep specialists can prescribe the non-surgical approaches. Ear, Nose, and Throat specialists and Oral Surgeons with interest in Sleep Apnea are there to help with the surgical undertakings.

Non-surgical Obstructive Sleep Apnea Treatment:

Q. Isn't there just a pill I can take or something?

No. Unfortunately there is not an easy answer. Even weight loss is not universally effective at resolving OSA. Just throwing oxygen at the problem isn't enough either. There are no medical solutions that work, yet. **(Veasey)**

Q. So how can I fix my Sleep Apnea?

Now for the hard truth... Sleep Apnea is most likely a life long condition. And you probably don't have a quick fix.

The severity determines your options for therapy. Unless you have really mild OSA we don't have universally acceptable, reliable, and easy remedies. Treatment is more about controlling the problem to prevent the medical consequences of Sleep Apnea. Given the stakes and the options, we almost always start with CPAP.

On the bright side, if your Sleep Apnea is treated your life is better. Imagine life without the daytime drowsiness that interferes with your work and family life. Going to work refreshed, focused, efficient, and with the stamina to finish the day is awesome. To have the energy to spend time with your family after work is more than meaningful. Quality of life is improved.

And while you may not feel this daily, minimizing your risk of heart attack, stroke, heart failure, and uncontrollable high blood pressure is kind of nice. This is a HUGE impact on the <u>quantity</u> of your life.

Q. What is CPAP?

What you didn't want to hear about!

Risk free and universally effective, a Continuous Positive Airway Pressure (CPAP) machine is our #1 therapy for most people with Sleep Apnea.

All sleep specialists know that most every newly diagnosed person with OSA dreads hearing those words. No one wants to sleep the rest of his or her life wearing a mask, tubing, and a humidifier (that requires nightly filling and maintenance) connected to an air pump.

But CPAP works. It is a very simple therapy. A mask covers your nose, and occasionally your mouth too. It connects via a hose to an air pump at the bedside. The pump pushes air under pressure into your airway. The air pressure keeps your throat open and unobstructed while you sleep. (Imagine blowing into a balloon with just enough pressure to just keep it open but not inflated.) An open throat means unobstructed breathing no matter how deeply you are asleep.

CPAP is a hard sell. The "Tom Cruise in Top Gun" analogy always falls flat in the office. More often patients come back with "Darth Vader" references. No it isn't sexy or cool. The mask takes a lot of getting used to, particularly in the beginning. However, with consistent effort and persistence most people adjust to how it feels and sleep easily. Successful long-term CPAP users get to the point where they feel uncomfortable <u>not</u> wearing the mask. It becomes so much apart of their sleep routine they can't sleep without it. Sleep medicine doctors hit a home run if their patients are "hooked" on CPAP! This is a good addiction, protecting you from the ravages of Sleep Apnea, which is the whole point.

One other important point: your insurance company typically does not consider paying for any other intervention unless CPAP is tried first. So unless you want to pay for a procedure out of pocket, which can be pretty pricey, this is your first step.

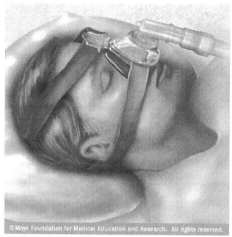

(Used with permission from "Continuous Positive Airway Pressure CPAP"
http://www.mayoclinic.org/
diseases-conditions/sleepapnea/multimedia/continuous-positive-
airway-pressure-cpap/img-20007977.)

Q. Isn't CPAP going to mess with my bed partner's sleep? I heard the machine is really loud.

Older CPAP machines were loud and huge. Modern digital technology has changed the game. The pumps and humidifiers are quiet. The whole set up hums gently, at worst like a white noise machine. Your bed partner will sleep in a MUCH quieter environment with CPAP working than during your life and death struggle with snoring and Sleep Apnea.

Q. What is a CPAP titration study?

Once you decide to give CPAP a try, your sleep medicine team needs to determine the pressure that effectively keeps your throat open and resolves your apnea. Except for the addition of the CPAP mask and set up, this night is the same as your diagnostic sleep study. Same place. Same monitors. But this time the sleep technician is actively involved in the study. He or she adjusts the CPAP pressure remotely from another room, starting low and increasing until the airway stays open, even on your back in REM sleep. Once the technician finds an effective pressure setting (which is measured for some reason in "centimeters of water") you get to sleep off the rest of the night. Your sleep doctor reads and interprets the study afterwards. Then the two of your decide if CPAP is the right answer for you. If we can get you treated in the lab, we can probably get you to sleep well at home.

Having a technician perform the pressure titration in the lab is beneficial for longer-term success. He or she is available to help before, during and after the study. An experienced professional can address all mask questions, comfort problems, expectations, and technical issues for you. And with their active assistance, finding a successful treatment is the usual outcome.

Q. What is a "Split Night Study"?

Two sleep studies (diagnostic and then therapeutic) is the "gold standard." But, if the diagnosis is fairly certain, the study may be ordered as a "Split Night." Patients and insurance companies like this approach. It is cheaper and more convenient to get it both diagnosis and treatment done at one time. And, doing it all in one sleep study gets you started on treatment sooner.

But, to qualify for a Split Night Study, you have to demonstrate real Sleep Apnea within the first two hours. Your apnea hypopnea index (AHI) has to be at least 40 events per hour, or between 20 and 40 events per hours WITH associated severe sleepiness, problems thinking/concentrating, heart disease, high blood pressure, or lung disease. If you meet these strict diagnostic criteria, the tech has plenty of time left in the night to titrate to your effective CPAP pressure. **(Kushida)**

There are a large number of these split night studies that become two night studies, though. If your apnea is not demonstrated early enough to prompt the pressure titration, a second night dedicated solely to CPAP titration is necessary.

71

Q. Can't I just do a home CPAP titration too? Is it as good as an in-lab titration study? My study in the lab didn't find an effective pressure.

If an in-lab titration study can't find a treatment level that works, you may need to return for another full night on the CPAP. Another option is to do it at home.

The approach is a little different than a diagnostic home study. Most modern CPAP machines have an automatic pressure titrating (AKA auto-titration) function that adjusts on the fly. The pressure varies according to need, delivering only what is necessary to keep your airway open. The machine is preset to provide a range of pressures from reasonably low to very high. Sensors within the machine detect airflow. When airflow stops the machine interprets this as an apnea or hypopnea. In response, air pressure is increased to break through the obstruction. When you are breathing comfortably the machine hovers at the lowest pressure that maintains regular airflow.

These amazing machines also store information about your sleep and the effectiveness of the CPAP. And no, you can't cheat by turning it on and setting it on the bedside table. The CPAP machine senses active breathing to determine hours of use nightly. (It knows when you've been sleeping, it knows when you're awake, it knows if you've been bad or good...)

Typically after a month or so, all of that information is gathered and downloaded into a program that gives your Sleep Medicine doc a pretty good idea of how you are doing. We know if you are struggling by how long and when you have worn it. We also get a reasonably good gauge of effectiveness. Most importantly, we see where the machine decided your pressure needed to be.

Often this hands-off approach is able to provide information about pressure effectiveness. And as a bonus, it does so while providing therapy.

Q. Do I really have to use CPAP?

CPAP is your safest, least invasive, and most effective treatment option. If you have an effective pressure that eliminates your Sleep Apnea you are set for healthier sleep. There is one catch:

you have to wear the $^%#*ing thing for it to work. Strapping a mask on your face every night, dealing with the equipment, cleaning it, getting new supplies, and interacting with your insurance company – for the rest of your life – is a real pain. It is disheartening. It is depressing. It is all those things. But CPAP works amazingly well.

Persistence and acceptance are keys to victory.

If CPAP is probably your only good choice, you have two options: 1.) Decide to be sleepy and suffer the long-term medical complications of untreated sleep apnea, or 2.) Take charge of your life and make this contraption work for you.

What Dr. B says to first time CPAP users?

No one wants to be on CPAP. I suspect that many people don't even bring up their sleep problems when they see their doc because they are afraid they may end up wearing one. Lots of people come to me with great anxiety just about the possibility of CPAP. They are stuck between feeling horrible because to their OSA and feelings of dread about having to wear something on their face to bed every night – forever. This is common, reasonable, and normal. But wearing CPAP is a lot better than what you are doing now.

CPAP disrupts your normal sleep routine. This is the hardest part. The nighttime ritual that helps you wind down and get ready to sleep is really important. You have some variation on tooth brushing, face washing, PJ wearing, pillow adjusting, and alarm setting that gets you ready for bed. Leave something out from, or add something into, this routine and it is harder to fall asleep. Strapping a mask around your head and blowing air pressure into your nose can be really disruptive.

This analogy may help explain how to adjust to the mask and machine. Imagine that you start wearing a SCUBA mask to bed. It is bulky, hot, you can't breath through you nose, and it hits the pillow every time your roll over…you would probably have trouble sleeping if you had it on. But, if a SCUBA mask cured Sleep Apnea, I bet you'd try. Eventually you would get used to wearing it. And you'd wake up every day feeling better and happier. Once you got used to it, if you didn't wear the SCUBA mask something would be amiss: your face would be cold, you could breathe through your nose, you just wouldn't feel right. You would probably have trouble falling asleep. And when you finally did, your sleep wouldn't be restful. The next day you would remember why you wore it in the first place.

CPAP is a lot better than a SCUBA mask! Initially it is so foreign and disruptive that you can't imagine wearing it to sleep. But given enough time you will adjust. That mask and its tubing become so much a part of your sleep you feel naked in bed without it.

No, your doctor can't force your compliance. The gun to your head is the consequences of not getting treatment for your apnea.

That is why I work really hard to help you succeed. There are a lucky few who strap on the mask and after one night say, "Wow, this is great!" Most people take a little more time and effort to get there. The best reward from CPAP is how you feel after 7 or 8 uninterrupted hours of sleep. If you haven't experienced that in a while, it is really awesome. Once you start feeling comfortable with the mask, and are lost without it, we have you hooked!

Q. What is Bilevel CPAP (BiPAP)?

This is CPAP's more serious cousin. Sometimes the CPAP setting is so high that you cannot exhale comfortably. The work-around is to lower the pressure on exhalation and ramp it back up on inhalation: thus "bi-level" pressure. Just like with CPAP the inhaled pressure is set high enough to keep the airway open. The exhalation pressure is lowered to make it easier to tolerate. Bi-level PAP and CPAP are equally effective at Sleep Apnea treatment. Comfort drives the decision for one or the other. During a CPAP titration if the pressure moves higher than around 14 the tech may switch to a bilevel setting. The goal is to find a pressure that is comfortable and effective.

Q. I have been told that I need to use a humidifier on my CPAP machine. Why?

Forced room air dries and congests the nose. A stuffy nose prevents effective transmission of air pressure to keep the throat open. Heated humidifiers fix that problem. Warm, moist, filtered air is much kinder to the nose. No dryness + no congestion = successful CPAP.

Q. Which mask is right for me?

That is completely a personal preference. There are bunches of different masks made by the sleep companies. None are perfect for everyone and none are universally acceptable. The mask that works best is the one that most comfortably fits your face.

Your nasal airway and the pressure setting on the machine also have an impact on which one to choose. Nasal "pillows" are popular as they are fairly small and not as disruptive. However, if the pressure is high, the "pillows" don't seal well enough. A nasal mask that provides a better seal is your best bet. If your nose is a mess and you are a mouth breather, a full-face mask can get you the pressure you need.

You will work with a durable medical equipment (DME) provider to figure out what works best for you. And they will keep your equipment up to date and working well.

Q. My nose is stuffy all of the time anyway. Can I use CPAP?

Your first visit with a sleep specialist should include a discussion of your nose. Can you breathe through it? Allergies an issue? Congestion during the day/night/always? What do you do to improve breathing? Medications, Breathe Rite® Strips, salt water nasal spray/wash? Does anything help? Nasal congestion makes OSA worse. So, if your nose is blocked we need to figure out why. If swelling and congestion is caused by stuff in the air (pollens, dust, smoke, etc.) topical anti-inflammatory/allergy medication is tried. These nasal steroids and antihistamines are safe and don't cause drowsiness. You have enough of that already.

If there is an anatomical obstruction, like a deviated septum and/or turbinate enlargement, you may need surgery to succeed with CPAP, discussed in more detail below.

Q. If my nose is messed up can't I just use a mask on my mouth instead?

If your nose a mess, medications aren't working, and you don't need/want surgery, a full-face mask covering the nose and mouth is an option. You may find it comfortable and do just fine. But, the size of the mask can be overwhelming and you might have trouble adjusting to it. Since it covers much of the face, you may feel claustrophobic with the full-face variety. But if it works for you it is the right one.

Q. What about the oral device that is supposed to fix Sleep Apnea?

The Mandibular Advancement Device (MAD) has its place in the right patient with OSA. It resembles upper and lower orthodontic retainers. A crank connects the 2 mouthpieces. Over time, the lower jaw is pulled progressively forward. This advancement also pulls the tongue and tonsil area forward and out of the airway. **(Hoffstein)**

Compared to CPAP, the MAD is fairly effective. CPAP is generally better at consistently improving apneas and oxygen levels over time. **(Doff)** But there are patients for whom this is an attractive alternative.

If you have a short jaw, a large tongue, mild sleep apnea, and just can't handle CPAP, the MAD may be for you. There are some occasional downsides to the MAD: jaw (TMJ or temporomandibular joint) problems, drooling, and dry mouth. **(Ontario Review)** I had a patient who needed braces after MAD. The pressure on the teeth pulled them out of alignment. These are all fortunately rare complications

Getting a dental device requires connecting with a dentist who knows what they are doing. It takes a special expertise and interest to do this right. They usually work with a medical sleep specialist as part of the treatment team. Finding an expert dentist minimizes your risks and maximizes your success.

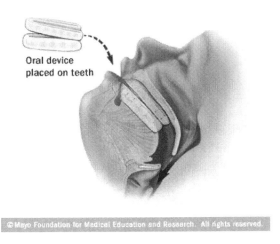

Oral device
placed on teeth

(Used with permission from "Obstructive sleep apnea."
http://www.mayoclinic.org/diseases-conditions/obstructive-sleep-apnea/multimedia/oral-device/img-20007681)

Q. My sleep doc told me that the only time I have sleep apnea is when I sleep on my back. My wife has been telling me this for a long time. Is there anything out there that fixes that?

Indeed there is. This approach can work great.

"Positional Therapy" simply keeps you off your back, the position that is most problematic for Sleep Apnea. REM-A-TEE® (antisnoreshirt.com) and ZZoma® (zzomaosa.com) both have belts that contain bumpers to prevent back sleeping. Both are FDA approved and available by prescription. REM-A-TEE also has a t-shirt that holds a small inflatable pillow in a pocket on the back. Same effect.

I once had a patient sew a tennis ball into the back of an old concert t-shirt one time. Whatever works for you.

Q. Can't I just lose weight and avoid all of this?

If only it were that easy! There are a few people are lucky and lose weight to fix their Sleep Apnea. If you are one of the lucky ones, terrific. It requires a total renovation in how you live your life. Regular exercise, wise diet decisions, and good sleep are at the core of the transformation. We often recommend CPAP as a short-run bridge until the weight is off. When you are at a healthy weight we can readdress whether you still really need the machine.

Weight Loss – Dr. B's Opinion

This is one of the most vexing parts of sleep apnea treatment. Weight is not the only risk factor, of course. But the heavier you are, the more likely you are to have Sleep Apnea. Also, being overweight is tightly linked with diabetes, high blood pressure, and heart disease. Those problems are bad enough. Untreated Sleep Apnea just makes them worse.

Weight loss is a very simple proposition at its core. You have to burn off more calories than you take in. There is nothing magic about it. Really. How you burn off those calories and what you eat is the challenge. My view is very simplistic:

Eat healthy foods in moderation. Increase physical activity.

I know this isn't groundbreaking information. But, this simple formula is how all weight loss efforts succeed. Victory comes through knowing what you need to change and finding a way to follow through.

I fervently believe that we eat too many prepared foods. We have lost touch, for the sake of convenience, with what we are really eating. We seem to have more important things to do besides caring about our food and health. Our time is better spent sitting in our car in the drive through or hanging out on the couch watching TV while the microwave "cooks" dinner. Notice the emphasis on sitting. We do a lot of that today.

Ironically, we have access to healthier, safer, fresher food than at any time in the history of the world. We have fresh fruits and vegetables available year round. Modern food handling and preparation techniques protect against food-borne illnesses. Our ancestors, even just 50 years ago, would be stunned to see the daily offerings in the grocery store. And still we go eat fast food and snack to extreme. Why?

One reason is taste. We like high fat, salty foods. Compare the taste of raw peanuts to honey roasted salted ones. I rest my case. It is hard to overcome the desire for a bacon double cheeseburger when all you have in front of you are carrot sticks. That is where will power and self control come in. Sure it is ok to indulge on occasion. Just make it the exception rather than the rule.

Another reason is cost. It is a lot cheaper and easier to eat at McDonalds than to buy and prepare the hamburger, buns, cheese, and condiments. The cost of ripe tomatoes, good ground beef, whole grain buns, pickles, and fresh lettuce is higher, in the short run than buying a fast food burger. Cooking frozen french fries in the oven isn't too hard, but they are soaked in oil so why bother? There are canned vegetables, canned fruits, and an enormous variety of frozen entrée's (not just pizza) waiting in the grocery store. Throw them in the microwave and dinner is served. Unfortunately, those premade foods are high in fat and salt and lack the nutritional power of "real" foods.

I read "The Ominvore's Dilemma" (**Pollan**) hoping to gain some insight into modern diets. The bottom line I gleaned from his book was this: "If you can afford to eat organic you should. It is probably healthier for you." I was a bit stunned at the lack of better ideas. If you have ever browsed your local "We Care About the World so Buy our Organic Produce and Dietary Supplements" market (Whole Foods, I'm looking at you) you probably had some sticker shock. It is insanely expensive to try to eat "right." It costs more to farm and raise livestock "organically and naturally." For most of us, eating air-chilled-free-range-grass-fed-shiatsu-massaged-read-to-nightly-high-self-esteem poultry is not really worth $8 a pound.

So what is my answer, you may be asking? It is simple. Eat smartly and within your budget. Have a wide variety of foods on your plate. Have something raw with every meal. Substitute fruit for dessert. Have a salad instead of fries. Go to Farmer's Markets and eat fresh food in season. Eat lean meats that are baked or broiled or grilled or boiled. Forego fried foods except on rare occasions. Have your coffee black without cream and sugar. Drink water instead of soda. And, if you can afford it, eat more fish and chicken. Don't worry too much about organic if the food is fresh. I'd rather you eat tomatoes off the vine than out of the can no matter where they came from.

And take the time to prepare your own food. Prioritizing sleep is a main theme in this book. Learn to prioritize your health.

Take charge of what goes in to your body by making your own dinner whenever you can. Make it a family affair. Involve your kids so that they develop healthy eating habits, too. Connect them with what goes into their meals so they can make good choices when they have families.

Finally, you have to be more active if this weight loss thing is going to happen. Eating differently is not enough. Get off the couch, turn off the TV and take a walk after dinner. It is free, highly effective, and a much better use of your time than seeing NCIS reruns, again.

Surgical Fixes (A.K.A. "Not CPAP") for Obstructive Sleep Apnea:

Q. Isn't there a surgery that can just fix my Sleep Apnea so I don't have to keep dealing with it?

Well kinda sorta…not really…sometimes…uh, maybe.

That is a difficult question to answer. It should be easy, right? There aren't that many places where a problem can occur. But treatment is more complicated than that. Surgical therapy for Sleep Apnea is not an exact science. It is difficult to accurately determine the site(s) of obstruction in every individual. There usually isn't a simple surgical cure.

Weight has a big impact. The projection of the face and jaw influences the position of the tongue and palate. The nose may be crooked and internally obstructed. Big tonsils may run in your family. You may have the longest uvula ever recorded. You may have some, or all, of these problems. It is difficult to know what part of each problem causes your unique Sleep Apnea issue.

Also, there is no guarantee that any surgical procedure always works on anybody. There is a place for surgery, no doubt. You need to approach any operation for Sleep Apnea with all of your options in front of you. Now do you see why we start with CPAP?

Q. How can I know if surgery is even a possibility for me?

Sit down and talk to your ENT or Oral Surgeon. He or she should be up front with you about your surgical options and the likelihood of success. In general, the more severe your apnea the less the likelihood of surgical cure. This is not meant to discourage you, as surgical cures happen. You need to be realistic about the outcomes you can expect.

At very least, operations should decrease severity. But what is the point of having surgery if you still have Sleep Apnea and still have to wear a CPAP mask? Why not just skip the painful part and head directly to the mask, right?

Bottom line: there is not a one-size-fits-all procedure that cures OSA.

Surgical Procedures

Even though I have just bashed the potential helpfulness of surgery, there are times when it is needed and very useful. So let's go through what is available, from the top down.

NOSE:
Problem: An obstructed nose contributes to throat collapsibility and snoring/apnea.
Cause: Allergy, nasal inflammation, or anatomical obstruction: deviated nasal septum and/or enlarged turbinates.
Treatment: Surgery is considered if medical treatment with allergy care and topical therapies are ineffective. Septoplasty - bent, twisted, or curved midline cartilage and bone is straightened to improve space for airflow.
Turbinate Reduction – enlarged and/or engorged structures on the sidewall of the nose are reduced to improve airflow.
Setting for the Procedure: Operating room, often under general anesthesia, usually outpatient.
Recovery: 10-14 days.

Pain Level: 4-6/10. Pain medications used for 3-5 days. Nasal congestion until the internal splints are removed 5-10 days later.

Risks: Bleeding (very uncommon), infection (extremely uncommon), continued nasal obstruction (due to continued deviation despite the surgery or allergies/environmental influences with continued swelling).

Septoplasty with Turbinate Reduction

Septum and **Turbinates**

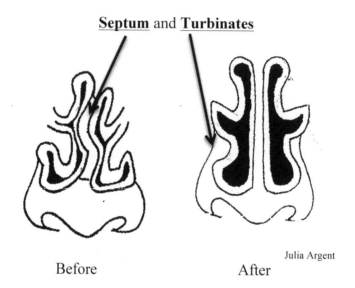

Julia Argent

Before   After

   Most people have Septoplasty and Turbinate Reduction solely for nasal congestion, not OSA. Quality of life is reliably enhanced due to improvement in the nasal airway, **(Naraghi)** which is nice. Doing this for OSA decreases nasal resistance to CPAP at very least. It also improves CPAP effectiveness and tolerance if needed. **(Camacho)**

ADENOID:
Problem: Swollen adenoid (tonsil-like) tissue obstructing the back of the nose, which contributes to snoring, throat collapsibility, and apnea.
Cause: Your natural adenoid size, infections, tumor

(extremely rare).

Treatment: Surgery is considered if the adenoid is confirmed to be obstructive, often by office nasal endoscopy.

Adenoidectomy –adenoid removal, approached through the mouth, opens the airway behind the nose to improve airflow.

Setting for the Procedure: Operating room, under general anesthesia, usually outpatient.

Recovery: 7-10 days. Pain

Pain Level: 4/10. May need a mild pain medication for sore throat.

Risk: Bleeding (extremely uncommon), continued Sleep Apnea.

<u>Adenoid</u>

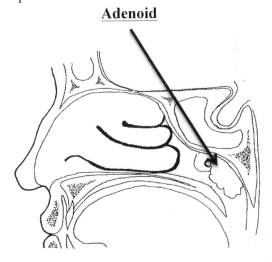

Julia Argent

Adenoid enlargement is very uncommon in adults, but it is worth evaluating as part of your overall assessment.

<u>PALATE:</u>

Problem: Redundant, excess tissue that narrows or hangs down at the back of the roof of the mouth – the soft palate. This collapsible area may flop around (snoring) or obstruct the airway (OSA).

Cause: Your natural palate size (most commonly).
Repetitive trauma from snoring and apnea can

induce swelling that compounds the problem.

Treatment: Surgery is considered if the palate is obstructive. Uvulopalatopharyngoplasty (UPPP) – Excess palatal tissue (and tonsils if present) is removed to open the back of the throat and the airway.

Setting for the Procedure: Operating room, under general anesthesia, usually with an overnight stay in the hospital.

Recovery: 14+ days.

Pain Level: 9-10/10. Severe pain requiring prolonged pain medication use – 10-14 days.

Risk: Bleeding (1%), continued Sleep Apnea, nasal regurgitation of liquids during swallow.

UVPP

| **Before** | **After** |

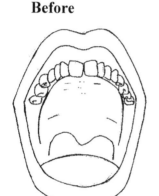 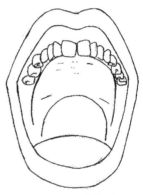

Julia Argent

That's right - you may endure this difficult procedure and still have sleep apnea. It is difficult to predict if UPPP will significantly reduce the severity of your Sleep Apnea. Cure is even more elusive. **(Caples)** At worst, it should decrease the severity of your OSA. If you have really mild sleep apnea your odds of cure are better.

TONSILS:

Problem: Large tonsils narrow the back of the throat, collapsing and obstructing the airway during sleep causing both snoring and/or OSA.

Cause: Your natural tonsil size (most commonly), recurrent infections, tumor (extremely rare).

Treatment: Surgery is considered if the tonsils are
obstructive.

Tonsillectomy - removes the obstruction.

Setting for the Procedure: Operating room, under general
anesthesia, occasionally with an overnight stay in the
hospital.

Recovery: 14 days.

Pain Level: 9-10/10 Severe pain requiring prolonged pain
medication use – 10-14 days.

Risk: Bleeding (1%), continued Sleep Apnea.

Tonsillectomy

Before   After

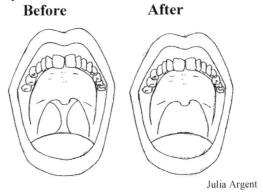

Julia Argent

Adults rarely have huge tonsils as the sole cause of OSA, but
it happens. Recovery is rough to say the least. If your tonsils could
eat Cincinnati you are a good candidate. There is very little scientific
data about the effect of tonsillectomy on OSA, though.

TONGUE, SURGERY:

Problem: Large tongue falls backward, obstructing the
airway during sleep causing snoring and/or OSA.

Cause: Your natural tongue size or jaw position does not
support the tongue forward and out of the airway.

Treatment: Surgery is considered if the tongue is visibly
obstructive. Often done as a component of a larger
operation that may include palatal surgery and
tonsillectomy.

Radiofrequency (RF) Tongue Base Reduction -
Burning the back of the tongue with a
radiofrequency energy probe shrinks and scars the

85

tissue, decreasing obstruction below the level of the palate.

Midline Tongue Reduction - Used for huge tongues, it involves the physical removal of tissue from the middle and back of the tongue.

Setting for the Procedure: RF Tongue Base Reduction is sometimes done under local anesthesia in an office setting as an outpatient procedure.

Midline tongue reduction, and RF if done as part of a multilevel surgery, usually performed in the operating room under general anesthesia, almost always with an overnight stay in the hospital.

Recovery: 14 days.

Pain Level: 8/10

Risk: Bleeding, short-term difficulty swallowing, continued Sleep Apnea

Radiofrequency Tongue Base Reduction

Before   After

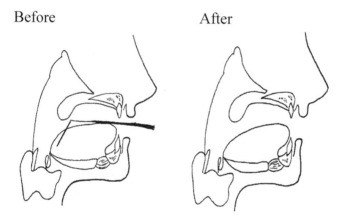

Julia Argent

Complete resolution of Sleep Apnea is unlikely with Radiofrequency Tongue Base Reduction alone. **(Aurora)** More aggressive tongue excision also does not reliably result in cure. **(Friedman, M)** Combining the RF procedure with UPPP (see above) does provide an additive effect to further decrease OSA severity. This approach is still unlikely to cure. **(Plzak)**

86

TONGUE, STIMULATION:

Problem: Large tongue falls backward obstructing the airway during sleep causing both snoring and/or OSA.

Cause: Your natural tongue size or jaw position does not support the tongue forward and out of the airway.

Treatment: People with moderate to severe OSA, who have failed CPAP, do not have a collapsing palate, and are not obese, may qualify for Hypoglossal (tongue nerve) Stimulation. **(Inspire®)** A battery-powered controller is implanted under the skin of the chest. Wires to chest muscles (below) and the nerve that moves the tongue forward (above) lead into the box. When the chest moves during a breath, the tongue is stimulated to thrust forward, moving it out of the throat and airway.

Setting for the Procedure: This is a multistage operation. First a sedated examination to determine the site of your airway collapse is done in the operating room. If the collapse is the NOT a circumferential collapse of the palate and isolated to the base of the tongue you may qualify. A second operation under general anesthesia is performed to implant the controller and wires.

Recovery: 10-14 days.

Pain Level: 6-8/10

Risk: Bleeding, infection, 3 scars, temporary or permanent tongue weakness, need for battery replacement (8-10 years down the road), continued Sleep Apnea.

Inspire

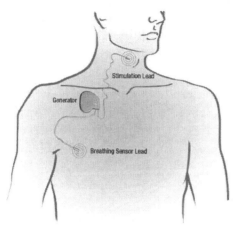

Image used with permission: Inspire Medical Systems

This is a big commitment. It is relatively new, but long-term tolerance is proven. **(Steward)** Effectiveness and applicability are still being worked out. Early indications indicate that it does seem to work as advertised and has fairly low surgical risk. **(Dehdhia)** Like all of these treatments, Inspire® may not cure Sleep Apnea. **(Strollo)**

TONGUE ADVANCEMENTS:

Genioglossus Advancement:
Problem: Large tongue base (back of the tongue) obstructs the airway during sleep causing both snoring and/or OSA.

Cause: Your natural tongue size or jaw position does not support the tongue forward and out of the airway.

Treatment: The genioglossus muscle attaches the front muscles of the tongue to the inside of the jaw. It is responsible for sticking the tongue out of the mouth. Pulling a window of bone to which the muscle is attached forward pulls the whole tongue forward – and out of the airway.

Setting for the Procedure: Operating room, often with an overnight observation stay.

Recovery: 10-4 days.

Pain Level: 7/10

Risk: Bleeding, infection, change in facial profile (which may be a positive in a person with a "weak chin"), swallowing problems, continued Sleep Apnea.

Genioglossus Advancement

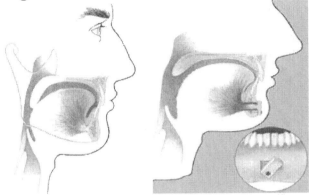

Used With Permission, Kasey Li, DDS, MD.
http://www.sleepapneasurgery.com/solutions_adults.html

HYOID ADVANCEMENT:

Problem: Large tongue base (back of the tongue) obstructs the airway during sleep causing both snoring and/or OSA.

Cause: Your natural tongue size or jaw position does not support the tongue forward and out of the airway.

Treatment: The hyoid is a horseshoe shaped bone situated above the voice box. It is an anchor for several muscles involved in swallowing, including some from the back of the tongue. Attaching this bone to the voice box, or the inside of the jaw, moves it and muscles at the back of the tongue forward and out of the airway.

Setting for the Procedure: Operating room, under general anesthesia, often with an overnight stay.

Recovery: 10-4 days.

Pain Level: 6-8/10

Risk: Bleeding, infection, swallowing problems, continued Sleep Apnea.

Hyoid Advancement

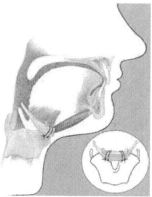

Used With Permission, Kasey Li, DDS, MD.
http://www.sleepapneasurgery.com/solutions_adults.html

Rarely are these two tongue advancement procedures performed as standalone operations. They are mostly part of multilevel surgeries that involve one or both tongue advancements and the palate (UVPP). In that setting, they is successful at reducing the level of sleep apnea. **(Yin)** Cure remains elusive with these procedures.

And if you thought those procedures were radical…

MAXILLOMANDIBULAR ADVANCEMENT:
Problem: Facial skeletal structure does not support the airway leading to collapse during sleep and snoring/sleep apnea.

Cause: The structural anatomy of your face.

Treatment: An extensive workup to measure and plan the facial rearrangement precedes the surgery. Orthodontia and braces are often part of the procedure. The surgery moves the upper and lower jaws forward, dragging the palate and tongue with them, thereby opening the airway. Titanium plates

securely fix the bones in place. This whole process
may take over a year to complete.

Setting for the Procedure: Operating room, under general
anesthesia.

Recovery: 14-21 days. Soft diet for weeks after the surgery.

Pain Level: 8/10

Risk: Bleeding, infection, bite misalignment, change in
facial contour, nasal obstruction, facial numbness,
continued Sleep Apnea.

Maxillomandibular Advancement

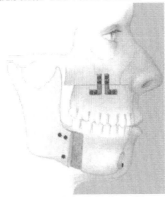

Used With Permission, Kasey Li, DDS, MD.
http://www.sleepapneasurgery.com/solutions_adults.html

This very invasive approach has the best results of all the
surgical therapies for Sleep Apnea. In the right person, the number
of breathing disruptions (AHI) is reduced by almost 90%. **(Caples)**
Not everyone is cured, but Maxillomandibular Advancement is our
most successful surgical intervention short of a Tracheotomy (see
below). Long term cure rates are excellent, if you are a candidate.
(Li)

Q. Am I a good candidate for those surgeries?

In general, the milder your Sleep Apnea the more likely that
surgery will help. The converse is equally true. Like everything in
life, nothing is 100%. There are plenty of people who have mild
sleep apnea who failed surgery and are on CPAP. There are also a
few people whose severe Sleep Apnea was cured surgically. To date,

this is an inexact science. It is very difficult to consistently define the exact combination of problems that leads to your particular brand of OSA. Everyone's anatomy is different and there is no way to always predict success on a person-to-person basis.

Your most important first step after diagnosis is to consult with an experienced ENT or Oral Surgeon with an interest and expertise in Sleep Apnea. A complete head and neck exam to evaluate your airway and a review of your sleep study determines if you are a reasonable surgical candidate.

Let me reiterate. No surgery can be counted upon to ALWAYS cure Sleep Apnea, no matter what that ad in the airline magazine might say. There are only two absolute certainties in the treatment of sleep apnea. 1.) CPAP/BiPAP will work for the overwhelming majority of people with OSA **if** they wear it; and 2.) A tracheotomy is the ultimate answer.

Q. What is a tracheotomy?

A plastic tube (called a trach tube) is placed surgically into the windpipe through the front of the neck. At night the tube is unplugged so that you breathe directly into the lungs, bypassing the obstructed nose, mouth, and throat. During the daytime you breathe around the plugged tube.

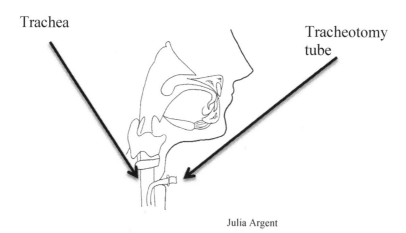

Trachea

Tracheotomy tube

Julia Argent

This is the ultimate answer to Sleep Apnea. No obstruction, no more apnea. It's that easy, sort of. A trach is huge intrusion into your neck and your life and a real hassle to care for. But it really works, if that is your only option.

Q. A trach tube? Really?

Of course you don't want this operation. No one does. But, occasionally it is necessary. Some Sleep Apnea is so bad that CPAP/BiPAP through a trach is needed. If you have Pickwick Syndrome (see page 62 for more information) – obesity, heart failure, dramatic daytime sleepiness, and impending demise if something is not done – a trach may be just the ticket.

Obviously, given the choice you would NOT want a trach. Unless there is a medical necessity or some other big time medical issue, CPAP is a much more attractive choice.

To summarize...

Surgical Sleep Apnea Therapies

Anatomical Site	Surgery
Nose	Septoplasty with turbinate reduction – Anatomical obstruction is removed to improve nasal airflow.
Adenoid	Adenoidectomy – Removal of obstructive adenoid tissue from behind the nose to open the airway.
Throat	Uvulopalatopharyngoplasty (UVPP) – Mid part of the palate is removed to open the airway. Tonsillectomy – Enlarged and obstructive tonsils are removed to open the throat and prevent collapse.
Tongue	Tongue Base Reduction – Radiofrequency (RF) Ablation or Midline Reduction of the Tongue Base decrease the size of the back of the tongue to move it out of the airway and prevent collapse. Tongue Stimulation – Inspire®, a battery operated stimulator that synchronizes inspiration with movement of the tongue forward and out of the airway. Tongue Advancement – Genioglossus and Hyoid Advancement both move the skeletal support of the tongue forward, pulling the tongue up and out of the airway.
Facial Skeleton	Maxillomandibular Advancement – Moving the upper (maxilla) and lower (mandible) jaws forward pulls the tongue and palate forward and out of the airway.
Trachea	Tracheotomy – A tube is placed through the neck into the trachea (windpipe). At night the tube is opened, bypassing the upper airway altogether and relieving obstruction.

The Reality of CPAP - How you can succeed.

Q. Okay. You convinced me to try CPAP. Now what?

Your doctor prescribes the whole set up through a durable medical equipment (DME) company who is contracted with your insurance carrier. Included in the prescription is your particular effective pressure that was determined by a CPAP titration sleep study or an auto-titration setting. Insurance clearance is not difficult if you have documented real Sleep Apnea. The DME company will contact you to arrange for a visit at their place, or yours sometimes, to introduce you to your new nighttime companion. Most importantly, they should educate you on the use and care of your new CPAP machine.

You then take your equipment home, put it on your bedside table, stare at it that first night, sigh deeply, and put on the mask. You will not be excited. In fact you <u>should be</u> somewhat disheartened and discouraged. The rest of your life is staring at you. Yes: you will wear this every night for the rest of your life. Don't despair. CPAP takes a lot of getting used to. But once you get 7 to 8 hours of uninterrupted sleep again, it will be apparent why you are wearing it.

There is a lucky minority who falls asleep, and awakens with a big smile that first morning after a full night of uninterrupted sleep. Most people take a long time to adjust to wearing the mask and breathing with the pressure. We sleep docs do a lot of cheerleading in the first few months to get you to accept the idea and become accustomed to your treatment. Our best selling point is that feeling you will have after you got good sleep - all night. If we can get you to that point, you win.

Q. None of those things sound very appealing to me. What if I do nothing?

First, you are exposing yourself and the people around you to the consequences of being chronically sleepy. This includes the risks of drowsy driving. You could hurt yourself, your passengers, and others on the road if your fall asleep and lose control of the car.

Second, your work and family life suffers. Being chronically tired makes you less productive and happy. And finally, not treating your OSA sets you up for a lifetime of medical problems (and bills) that you might be able to prevent.

So you can choose to live in denial or you can take control of your life and do something to feel better. Up to you.

Q. OK already, you convinced me. How often should I see my sleep doctor when I am successful at CPAP usage?

In my practice I see you 1 month after starting the CPAP machine and then monthly thereafter until we have success. Then I see you at 6 months to check on your longer-term success. If all is well I will see you yearly thereafter.

I do long term follow up for two reasons. 1.) It is good medicine. I like to confirm that your sleep therapy is effective and you are healthy; and 2.) Insurance companies are increasingly requiring a physician's statement confirming successful CPAP use. Understandably they don't want to continue to pay for something if it is gathering dust in your closet.

Q. I have Sleep Apnea and have gained a lot of weight. My wife/husband says I am snoring again even with the mask on. What should I do?

Things change over time, including weight. It is possible that weight gain worsens apnea. Your current pressure may be insufficient to treat your new situation.

First, visit your DME provider to make sure the machine is still working correctly. If that is okay, see your Sleep Medicine doctor to reevaluate your sleep. You may need a repeat CPAP titration study (or a month-long auto-titration at home) to determine a new effective pressure.

Q. I am a professional driver with Sleep Apnea. I am required to take another sleep study even though I wear my CPAP all of the time. What is the Maintenance of Wakefulness Test (MWT) and why is it required?

The MWT is a measurement of your wakefulness. Your employer may want to confirm that your Sleep Apnea is successfully treated before allowing you back on the jobsite. It is a safety thing, for you and others. This test confirms that your CPAP therapy keeps you awake and alert.

Here is how the test goes.

1. You do an overnight sleep study with CPAP. This insures you have enough normal sleep to be adequately rested for the next day.
2. You get up, get dressed and have breakfast. The monitoring equipment that measured your sleep the night before stays on for the rest of the day.
3. You have 4 opportunities for "naps." You sit comfortably on the bed in a dimly lit and very quiet sleep lab bedroom. You have 40 minutes to try to stay awake. Yes, there is a break for lunch.
4. If you do fall asleep we wake you up after 90 seconds. Then, you get to wait another couple hours for the next "nap."

Almost 100% of normal sleepers are able to stay awake in this environment for 8+ minutes. If you average less than 8 minutes of awake-time during these 4 nap opportunities, you are not sleeping well enough and we have some work to do. You may have another sleep issue, a medical problem, or need for medication to keep you awake despite adequate treatment of your Sleep Apnea.

Q. What if I am sleeping well with my CPAP but am still sleepy during the day?

Up to 5% of people successfully treated with CPAP have continued daytime sleepiness. This may be a consequence of brain changes after years of sleep disruption due to OSA. If there is no other reason for your sleepiness (like another sleep diagnosis, a medical problem that disrupts sleep, or lack of sufficient hours of sleep) you may try a prescription "wake-promoter" medication. Nuvigil® (modafinil) or Provigil® (armodafinil) help you to stay awake safely and effectively. **(Inoue)**

Q. I have been on CPAP for months. I use it every night. I don't feel at all different. I thought this was supposed to change my life, right?

Unfortunately, some people on CPAP don't have a "sun finally came up" reinvigoration of their lives. Despite having real Obstructive Sleep Apnea effectively treated with CPAP there is no palpable change in how they feel during the day. This is a tough sell for the Sleep Medicine doctor.

Despite your lack of subjective improvement, CPAP is still doing you good. Giving your heart a rest from the ravages of repeated apnea should improve the QUANTITY of your life, even if your QUALITY has not changed much. Also, the quality of your bed partner's sleep has to improve in the absence of the racket you make without the machine. So there are positives, just not what you hoped for perhaps. Hang in there. It is worth it in the end.

Chapter 6: Central Sleep Apnea

"We all have different reasons for forgetting to breathe."
Andrea Gibson

Central Sleep Apnea refers to the brain (Central) forgetting to breathe (Apnea). This is clearly not the usual state of affairs. The brain is remarkably good at making sure all of our bodily functions work the way they are supposed to on a daily basis, minute by minute, second by second.

The breathing regulation control center lives in the brainstem. It senses tiny changes in the amount of oxygen (breathe in the good air) and carbon dioxide (breathe out the bad air) in the blood stream. As oxygen drops and carbon dioxide increases the brain's respiratory center sends a message to the lungs to get to work and move some air.

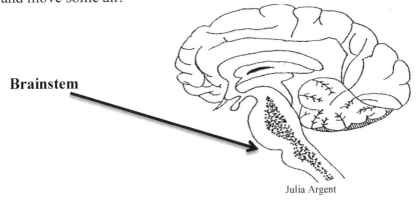

Brainstem

Julia Argent

Normally this finely tuned system keeps your breathing just right. But on occasion the breathing control center malfunctions as a result of head or brain injury, heart failure, a congenital brain malfunction, an overdose on a medication, or a rare genetic syndrome. Despite how horrible this sounds, Central Sleep Apnea is uncommon and rarely life threatening.

Q. What is Arnold Chiari Malformation?

This is an abnormality of the skull and brainstem. The foramen magnum (impressive name, huh?) is the big hole in the base of the skull through which the spinal cord passes as it leaves the brain. (See the picture above.) Some people are born with an abnormality that allows the back of the brain to shift down through the foramen magnum putting pressure on the brainstem. Headaches, incoordination, hoarseness, dizziness, ringing in the ears, and swallowing problems are typical initial complaints. Because the breathing control centers are in the brainstem, apnea (obstructive, central, or mixed central and obstructive) may also occur.

An MRI confirms the diagnosis. If the malformation is severe enough to cause symptoms, an operation is necessary to release pressure on the brainstem. It is a very big surgery, but it can save your life!

Q. How does Heart Failure cause Central Sleep Apnea?

Good question. It doesn't seem that these two should be related, but they can be.

First, heart failure means just what it sounds like. The heart fails to efficiently pump blood. Poor circulation leads to fluid accumulation in the lungs. Stiff, fluid filled lungs don't work very well and do a poor job of letting oxygen (O_2) in and carbon dioxide (CO_2) out. Sluggish circulation delivers blood slowly to the brain. Over time, chronic low oxygen and high carbon dioxide dulls the responsiveness of the brainstem breathing control center. Chaos results.

Central Sleep Apnea due to heart failure has a very typical breathing pattern. It goes like this...

Sluggish blood circulation to the lungs = low O_2, high CO_2.
↓
Brainstem notices late.
↓
Brainstem overreacts and breathing gets faster and faster.
↓
O_2 increases + CO_2 decreases.
↓
Brainstem stops breathing due to an over correction of the problem with high CO_2 and low O_2.
↓
O_2 decreases + CO_2 increases because breathing has stopped
↓
Brainstem overreacts: breathing gets faster and faster.
↓
And so on…. you are always playing catch up.

This repeating cycle of Hyperpnea - ("Hyper-" means excessive and "-pnea" refers to breathing) and Apnea ("A- means no and –"-pnea" refers to breathing) is called Cheyne-Stokes Breathing. (**Malhotra**) It has a classic graphical pattern. Check it out below.

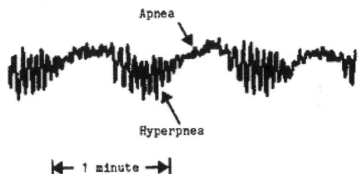

Treating the failing heart is the ultimate answer. Supplemental oxygen is helpful, especially if Cheyne-Stokes occurs along with lung disease. CPAP seems to help, too. Adaptive Servoventilation (see below) is probably the best option. (**Brown**)

Q. Do people breath like that after a stroke, too?

Anything that affects the brainstem breathing control center can cause Central Sleep Apnea. Cheyne-Stokes respirations also sometime occur after stroke, head injury, as an effect of some brain tumors, and with brainstem lesions due to multiple sclerosis.

Q. Do some people who overdose on drugs stop breathing?

Yes. "Narco" in Greek means stupor or numbness. Overdosing on a narcotic - like heroin - stops breathing and causes Central Sleep Apnea – permanently. Bad idea. Even when prescribed legally for legitimate pain control, narcotic medications can cause problems with sleep. Morphine (named after Morpheus, the Greek god of dreams), Methadose® (methadone), Percocet® (oxycodone), codeine, and Norco®/Vicodin® (hydrocodone) are all effective pain meds that can also cause significant daytime sleepiness. Because they depress brainstem breathing control centers at higher doses, Central Sleep Apnea is also possible.

Q. Is it possible to have both Obstructive and Central Sleep Apnea?

Yes. It is called Complex Sleep Apnea. Having a few central apneas during a sleep study is common, especially if you have really severe OSA. Multiple central apneas make life a little more complex. Adaptive Servoventilation (ASV) is a CPAP protocol that addresses both the obstructions and central events. ASV adapts its pressure to your need.

There are two approaches: 1.) Air volume support and 2.) Breathing rate support.

During a central apnea, the volume approach swells air through the mask and your airway to support and maintain it, thereby moving some air into the lungs. It is very effective.

The other method is to provide positive pressure breaths when needed. The machine senses the number of breaths you take per minute. If there are fewer breaths than a preset required rate, the machine pushes a breath into you, just like a ventilator.

Both approaches are useful and effective.

Q. So my Mom uses Google way too much and she thinks that I might have Congenital Central Hypoventilation Syndrome (CCHS) because I stop breathing at night. I tell her that it is just my Sleep Apnea and I'm not going to die. I'm right aren't I?

She needs to give up her MD from Google University!

Imagine holding your breath and not feeling panicked to inhale after a minute or two. That is how you feel if you have CCHS. This is a rare genetic disease associated with specific mutation (PHOX2B). This gene defect causes faulty brainstem oxygen and carbon dioxide sensors. While awake, breathing is fairly regular. When asleep, breathing can just stop.

This most often fatal problem runs in families and is usually diagnosed in childhood. Remarkably, though, some adults have a mild form of CCHS that is recognized later in life. Mortality rate is high unless it is treated early with a nighttime ventilator. **(Patwari)**

But it sounds like you just need to go get your sleep study!

Section 4: Sleep Timing Problems

"If I was to go to sleep before midnight, I would feel weird about myself, like I wasted a day. My most productive hours are between midnight and five."
J. Cole

Chapter 7: Circadian Rhythm Disorders

The daily cadence of life is not set by the cable TV schedule. We have a tempo, called the Circadian Rhythm, which influences just about everything our bodies do. This term, "circadian," means around ("circa") the day ("dian"), very descriptive. Circadian control is found in our DNA. "Clock genes" coordinate our wake/sleep patterns and activities with the day/night pattern of our world. If we were nocturnal, like a bat, our schedule would be inverted.

Circadian rhythms regulate more than just sleep function. Clock genes are active in all cells and organ systems. Hormones that control metabolism are synchronized for greater utilization of energy during the daylight than at night. And your behavior mirrors that schedule: you eat during the day and are comfortable fasting at night, coordinating your food consumption when you need it. **(Huang)** Body temperature fluctuates with the clock: warmest in the early evening and coolest in the early morning hours. Blood pressure varies with the Circadian rhythm, dropping at night and increasing during the day. Even lung function varies throughout the day.

The internal clock controls a lot of our lives.

There are two very important influences on the internal clock, light and Melatonin. Special receptors in the eye detect morning and evening light. Those receptors are connected to nerves that transmit that information to the part of your brain that controls your internal schedule. In the morning, as the sun rises, your brain wakes up. Decreasing light in the evening, usually between 7:30 to 9:30PM, triggers release of Melatonin. This hormone signals to your brain that it is time to wind down and sleep. **(van Geijlswijk)** Each day your internal clock is "reset" and synchronized to the light dark-cycle of the sun.

Normally your circadian rhythms are in sync with the rest of the world's timetable. You get up and go about the same time as everyone else. But it doesn't always work out that way.

Problems may arise if a person's intrinsic schedule is misaligned rom the rest of society. If you are an extremely late night or extremely early morning person, it may be difficult to fit your life into the dominant work and school schedule. And, there are two new sleep problems that occur due to the "jet-age" and the "we-work-all-of-the-time-in-the-name-of-productivity-era." Jet Lag and Shift

Work Syndrome occur because of how we live this modern life.

There are medical consequences to the disruption of the Circadian coordination of your life. Sleep deprivation due to shift work is linked to obesity and Type 2 diabetes. **(Prasai)** Heart disease is more common if blood pressure does not decrease at night. **(Routledge)** Lung disorders, like asthma, are worse after the sun goes down, too. **(Cattarall)** Obesity, high cholesterol, diabetes, and other, now common, medical problems are influenced by sleep, timing of food ingestion, and other normal physiologically "scheduled" bodily functions. **(Huang)** Healthy sleep can make a difference for many of these problems.

Q. Help me please. I can't get to sleep before 3:00 AM. I never did well in school because I always fell asleep in class. I am not an idiot but I can't keep a day job because I am so sleepy. What is wrong with me? Can you fix me?

You are, in sleep medicine jargon, a Night Owl. The proper name for your diagnosis is Delayed Sleep Phase Syndrome (DSPS). Your normal sleep time is <u>delayed</u> relative to the rest of the world. This is not a lifestyle choice or the grumblings of an adolescent who doesn't want to get up on a school day morning. Your clock is set differently, later, than most everybody else. If your normal sleep period is from 3:00AM to 11:00AM, but school and work start at 8:00AM, you are out of sync with the rest of the world. Sure, you can get up and shake off the cobwebs and work, but your body is programmed to be asleep until everybody else's lunchtime. By the afternoon, you are great. On the weekend when everyone else is pooped out and headed home from the club, you are still ready to party. As the bars close you are just hitting your stride. Trying to adjust your schedule to match everyone else's doesn't work well. If you go bed earlier than what your internal programming demands, you stare at the ceiling, toss, and turn.

You have an uncommon and discouraging problem. Delayed Sleep Phase Syndrome is frequently treated as Insomnia unless someone takes the time to figure it out. Often you are labeled lazy, unmotivated, and apathetic which is unfair and damages your chance to succeed in life. You are wired differently, not a loser. Misdiagnosis and frustration are the rule.

So what can you do? It is almost impossible to permanently change your internal clock's timing. Manipulating you (with medication) and your environment (with sleep timing and light exposure) to shift your sleep period earlier takes a lot of effort and perseverance. It can work, but is a lifelong struggle.

Melatonin

This hormone is an important sleep signal messenger, normally produced at the end of the day in response to decreasing light. It tells the brain to begin the wind down. Your melatonin production is delayed, which is one reason your "go to sleep" signal is much later compared to "normal." Melatonin is available as an over-the-counter sedative on the supplement aisle. Taking it in the early evening helps to sync your timing with everyone else's. Take half of a 1mg Melatonin pill around 9 PM - the time a "normal" person starts to get sleepy – which happens to be 3 to 6 hours before your normal late night bedtime. This approach works, but not very well. Low dose Melatonin can shift your bedtime only about 40 minutes earlier than your usual. **(van Geijlswijk)**

Sleeping Pills

Using a sedative to knock you out is not effective, either. Taking sleeping pills does not shift your internal sleep timing. It just knocks you out. So taking a medication alone is not going to do it.

Chronotherapy

Resetting your internal clock is called, appropriately enough, Chrono- (or time) therapy. It requires a complete reordering of your sleep. While sleep deprivation sounds like cruel and unusual punishment, it is a useful tool to get your sleep reset toward "normal."

If you are willing to stay awake until you are so tired that you fall asleep whenever you get the chance, we have an opportunity to change your intrinsic schedule. You start by going to bed 3 hours LATER than your normal bedtime for a few days. If your intrinsic bedtime is 3 AM, staying up until 6 AM is exhausting. After a couple of days your bedtime moves forward to 9 AM, again for 2 more days. This 3 hours advancement occurs every 2 days until you are going to bed at 10 or 11 PM. During this transition, you must

107

simulate normal light and dark circadian rhythm conditions. That means avoiding bright light exposure during those daytime "bedtimes." Blocking out all light when bedding down for the "night" makes a big difference in the brain resetting process.

The whole process takes about 2 weeks during which your work and family schedules get all mixed up. But if you successfully reset your clock go to bed at 11:00PM and awaken at 7:00AM refreshed and ready to go, we have hit a home run. Chronotherapy doesn't always work. Success requires a persistent, lifelong, effort on your part to maintain the schedule. **(Barion)**

Light Therapy

Exposure to really bright early morning light has the potential to shift your clock earlier. This approach requires two hours of sunlight (ideally) or a medical light bank every morning starting around 6 AM. Maintaining this schedule is difficult. You really need two full hours every day. There are no weekend breaks or vacation days from the light. Any deviation from the plan will return you to your old schedule. The light treatment may conflict with your work or family schedules as well. It is also expensive. A medical grade light bank may not be covered by insurance. Despite all of the difficulties, if you follow the plan you likely will feel better rested in the morning and will be better able to comply with a more "normal" schedule. **(Chesson)**

Therapeutic Reality

These approaches are all only partially effective on their own. Putting all of these ideas together under the guidance of a Sleep Medicine specialist is the usual treatment plan. Start with Melatonin just to see how far you get with the simplest approach. Ongoing Melatonin use helps with schedule maintenance, too. If you are really motivated, initiate a sleep deprivation protocol and then use light therapy once your schedule is better aligned.

You have to be doggedly persistent to succeed. You can't revert back to your old ways on the weekends and expect to be on track for Monday morning. You have to be disciplined and rigid with the new schedule for the rest of your life to be consistently readjusted.

Or, here is another very valid idea…Embrace Your Difference

Simply accept your schedule and adjust your life to it. Many people who are Night Owls gravitate to professions and lifestyles that allow them to sleep healthfully and be productive. Working from home, late night shifts, and self-employment (where you can set your own hours) are all justifiable accommodations to your normal. You may not fit into a conventional schedule like most people, but you can be happy and productive and fulfilled on a different timetable.

Q. I feel like I am missing out on the world. No matter what I do I can't stay awake past dinnertime. And then I am up in the middle of the night. What can I do?

You have Advanced Sleep Phase Syndrome (ASPS). Believe it or not "Morning Lark" is the term used in scientific journals to describe your sleep. "Morning Person" sounds better to me. No matter what you call it, when you have ASPS your normal sleep time is advanced, <u>earlier</u>, than most people. Just like with Delayed Sleep Phase Syndrome (see the question above), your preferred time to sleep is out of sync with the rest of the world. This is not a lifestyle choice. Your internal clock is set differently. Your normal sleep period starts in the early evening and ends in the early morning. Going to bed at 8:00PM and awakening at 3:00AM means a good and normal night's sleep for you. Unfortunately, work starts at 8:00AM. By the time afternoon rolls around your body is starting to wind down to get ready for bed. Sure, you can try to go to bed later but you probably will still awaken in the early morning. That is what your internal clock is telling your body to do.

A Morning Person can easily sync a productive schedule with the rest of the world. You can be at work during your wake period and function well. Socially you are at a significant disadvantage. After work get-togethers, parties on the weekends, dinners out, all conflict with the time your body says, "sleep."

The conventional wisdom is that the elderly are more often Morning Larks. Think of the old folks home with a "Blue Plate Special" dinner at 4:30 and lights out at 8:30. ASPS can affect anyone at any age, though.

Because this is not such a disruptive problem, there is not a lot of research in shifting the Circadian Rhythm of a Morning Person. Light therapy, chronotherapy (moving your bedtimes back until they correspond to "normal" sleep hours), and melatonin have all been studied. But there is no evidence that any of these therapies are very effective. **(Dodson)**

So what to do? Usually, not much. Your best answer is to adjust your life to your natural rhythm. Inform your family, friends, and work about your particular quirk and help them help you with your schedule.

Q. I have to travel for work. I mean really travel. I cover many miles, continents, and even oceans every time I am on a plane. I am so tired when I get to my destination, and when I get home for that matter, that I am not enjoying the trips or being very productive on either end. How can I get to sleep, wake up refreshed, and perform well when I am in a different time zone from home?

You suffer from "Jet Lag Syndrome." (Always add "syndrome" to something to make it sound official.) This problem is a consequence of modern travel. Jet Lag has only been in existence since the 1940s when transcontinental and transoceanic flights became possible. Columbus had no difficulties with his internal clock during his trip across the Atlantic. It took him about 11 weeks. When you fly from Madrid to Miami you have crossed the same number of time zones in 7 hours that Columbus did in almost 3 months. He adjusted as he went. You have to adjust to the new time at your destination on the fly. At max, you will naturally adjust only about 1 - 2 hours per day. **(Eastman)**

There are no magic potions or maneuvers that automatically sync your internal clock to your new time zone. But I can supply you with some ideas and strategies that make the transition easier and faster.

DOMESTIC TRAVEL

West to East

Travel toward the East from the Pacific Time Zone is much more difficult than the other direction. If your L.A. bedtime is usually 11 PM, you will feel like going to bed in New York around 2 AM. Waking up in New York at 7 AM is really at 4 AM in LA on your internal clock. Imagine preparing for an 8 AM business meeting in New York. That early in the morning (5 AM back home) may not be your best time of the day for critical thinking.

So how do you manage to be your best and well rested for a West to East trip? I can offer several ideas that may help: adjust your clock before you go, use supplements, and adjust your meeting schedule.

Prepare for your trip to the East Coast by adjusting your sleep schedule for a few days before the trip. Going to bed earlier (without light exposure) in the early evening and waking up early (with lots of light exposure) mimics the Eastern Time Zone. While it may not be convenient to schedule your sleep this way, it does prepare your internal clock for your destination.

Melatonin can help. Taking 0.5 – 5 mg Melatonin tablets (sold as an over-the-counter supplement) in the late afternoon/early evening for a week or so before the trip helps to set your clock to an earlier, East Coast, bedtime. **(Prasai)**

Caffeine seems to help too. It helps to maintain awareness and sharpens thinking skills when you are tired, which is an obvious benefit. But your morning cup of Joe makes a difference even beyond the wake up jolt you normally experience. Caffeine also has benefits in somehow helping to shift your internal clock. **(Sack)**

I have a couple of logistical suggestions also. Schedule an early morning flight so you have all day on the ground to adjust. Also, don't schedule important meetings/work responsibilities/fun activities early the next morning on your west to east jaunt. Know that you will do better later and adjust the agenda accordingly. Common sense planning makes sure you are on top of your game, especially if it is a short trip.

Jet Lag Prevention: Five Tips for West to East Domestic Flights:

1. Prepare days in advance if your trip is that important.
2. Try going to bed (in the dark) and waking up (in bright light) on the East Coast time schedule for 3 or 4 days before you go to adjust ahead of time.
3. -Melatonin at dusk Eastern Standard Time for a few days before you leave may set the table for you adjustment during your trip.
   -Melatonin at dusk when you get to the east coast helps you get to sleep earlier and adjust more quickly.
4. Judicious use of caffeine to clear the cobwebs in the morning is certainly allowed. Avoid it later in the day so you can get to sleep earlier on the local schedule.
5. Take an early flight and make sure that the meeting timetable at your destination is adjusted to your schedule so you can be at your best when needed.

East to West

Going East to West is a piece of cake. As a New Yorker, you will be ready to work earlier than your California hosts. Makes you look like a superstar! However, at night you will be tired earlier, so socially you may be at a bit of a disadvantage.

INTERNATIONAL TRAVEL

"Jet lag is Insomnia you are lucky enough to have in Europe." Unnamed FDA medication reviewer.

International travel is even worse than domestic. Let's say you live in Chicago and are travelling to London for a business trip, a seven hour time difference. Your overnight direct flight from

112

O'Hare to Heathrow takes off at 7:00PM, which is 2:00AM local time in London. Nine hours later you land in England as lunchtime approaches. The Londoners are looking forward to their ploughman's and a pint. You, on the other hand, are feeling like 4:00AM in Chicago. Even if you slept the entire flight your body is set for Central Standard Time, not Greenwich Mean Time, no matter what your watch might be telling you.

There is no way to instantly get onto local time. An adjustment of about 1 to 2 hours a day is what your body can naturally accomplish. **(Eastman)** The question is how best to adapt as quickly as possible to the local time zone so you can feel rested, productive, and enjoy the trip.

I contend that the more sleep you can get on the flight the better. More sleep makes you more rested and more able to function when you hit the ground. Your clock may be off, but at least you won't be sleep deprived, too. Getting sleep on the plane is not always that easy though.

Some people are like my Uncle Ed – the lights go out (or not) and you are asleep. No matter where or when. For the rest of us, it is a little tougher. A couple of suggestions are in order to make it easier on the plane. First, on the flight over try not to drink too much alcohol. It is hard to say no to that second or third glass of wine on an international flight. But, too much alcohol disrupts the quality of your sleep. Sleeping pills do the same thing. Hangovers are common with both booze and sedatives. But if you need to take something, a very short acting sleeping medication like Ambien® (zolpidem) can help. Second, minimize light exposure. Wear a sleep mask to create your own darkness. Now go to sleep.

Assuming you are as well rested as possible when you get there, you need to get adjusted as quickly as possible. Right off the bat, synchronize all of your activities to the local schedule, including meals. Food intake and energy utilization are under circadian control along with sleep and wake cycles. So taking your meals at the normal local times may help you body and metabolism adjust more quickly to the new time zone. **(Huang)**

Live the local schedule immediately, including the dark and light cycles of night and day. Expose yourself to bright early morning outdoor light on Day 1 of your trip. As dusk falls and it is getting dark, get ready for bed. Don't take naps or sleep at any daylight hour; this delays the adjustment period and messes with your nighttime sleep. Native light and dark exposure influences your adjustment speed.

Timing your meals and sleep definitely helps your body naturally accommodate to a new time zone. But 1 to 2 hours of adjustment a day still means almost a week before you have completely reset to the London schedule.

To be on top of your game as soon as possible you need to call in some outside assistance. Melatonin is the your best bet to get on track. Taking melatonin just before bedtime (at dusk preferably) increases your rate of adjustment by up to 30%. **(Sack)** That means that you are comfortable and sleeping well for a much longer portion of your trip.

Caffeine somehow speeds up your adjustment to the new time zone. **(Sack)** It also provides better wakefulness until you catch up to your host's schedule. **(Beaumont)**. Hitting the coffee shop in the morning and at lunchtime to keep your eyes open is a convenient way to achieve the effect. Make sure not to drink too much coffee too late in the day. Excessive caffeine can disrupt your nighttime sleep and delay your adjustment. **(Sack)**

Jet Lag Prevention: Five Tips for International Flights

1. Sleep on the flight over, as much as possible.
2. Do not overindulge on the flight; too much alcohol is bad. If you take a sleep aid, take one that has a <u>very</u> short duration (like Ambien®/zolpidem). And don't mix it with alcohol.
3. Immediately incorporate the rhythms of your destination into your life, including meals and light exposure.
4. Melatonin at sundown helps you adjust faster.
5. Judicious caffeine use keeps you more alert during the day (and may help you adjust more quickly). Be careful not to use it too late in the day.

One final thought…if you are taking long distance, short

duration trips for work (say a 2 day jaunt to London for a meeting) you might consider just staying on your home sleep schedule. It will be out of sync with your destination. And you will need to limit light exposure during your "night" if it doesn't correspond to local darkness. But for a couple of days, since it is impossible to adjust anyway, why not just keep your watch set to back home? Adjust your work schedule accordingly.

Q. I have a lot of problems because of night shift work. I am tired all of the time no matter what I do, at work and at home. What can I do to sleep well with this kind of schedule?

There is a name for your problem: Shift Work Syndrome. Lots of people work off-hour shifts. The 24 hour economy drives world class productivity. But there is a price to pay for the worker. An estimated 10% of people who do evening and night shift work have problems with their sleep. **(Drake)** Older workers struggle more. No matter the age, everyone who suffers from Shift Work Disorder is at greater risk for drowsy driving accidents, absenteeism, and personal problems.

Nurses are the classic case for rotating night shift work. Hospitalized patients require 24 hour, onsite, hands on, nursing care. How the work schedule plays out varies from place to place. Some hospitals have a permanent night shift and some rotate the night shift among their personnel. Regardless of how they are organized, this schedule is disruptive to everyone's sleep rhythms. Even if you are assigned a permanent night shift, complete adaptation to that schedule almost never occurs. Your ability to tolerate the shifts improves over time, though.

Also, if you are working at night you may have a family or friends who don't. Your familial or social responsibilities don't respect your need for daytime sleep. For instance, if you get home from your 8 hour shift at 7:00AM you may be the one responsible for getting the kids to school by 8:00AM. You may also have people awake in the house during the day, living their lives, while you are trying to get some shut-eye in preparation for the next night shift. Socially, this schedule can be very disruptive as well. Getting together with friends on the weekend is usually not well coordinated with your work schedule. So your life forces you to move back and forth from day to night sleeping even if you are permanently on the late shift.

Q. So what do I do to make it through these night shifts?

There is a lot of research into Shift Work Disorder. Why? Because sleepiness can significantly impact productivity and safety in industries that require this sort of schedule. In healthcare, the military, or the transportation industry sleep disruption and problems with wakefulness can result in death. So this is a serious topic. As of yet there are no definitive answers for avoiding the downsides of sleeping with a turbulent work schedule. There are some strategies that make sense and seem to help

If you are going to work when you should be asleep, get some rest right before your shift. A short nap is improves mental focus. It doesn't replace a full sleep period, but a nap provides some rest for your brain before making it work when it doesn't want to.

There are not too many work sites/situations where a therapeutic light bank is available to illuminate workers. But exposure to bright light early in the night shift may help with wakefulness and work effectiveness. If you can get some bright light exposure early in the night shift it also helps you sleep during the day when you are home.

After your shift, avoid bright light on your way home. And when you get there, make sure you sleep in a very dark, quiet environment. Dark sunglasses or goggles (as silly as that might sound) can keep the morning light from triggering that "WAKE UP SUNSHINE!" message from your biological clock. Sleeping in a dark room helps to keep you that way.

Melatonin might help, too. Taking it on the way to bed in the morning after your night shift helps you sleep. Taking a short-acting sedative is helpful if you can't get to sleep.

Finally, use supplements and/or medications to help keep you awake when you are at work. Caffeine, in the form of coffee, tea, or a pill, helps keep you alert and focused during your night shift. Timing, like usual, is everything. Caffeine late in the shift during the early in the morning hours may keep you from sleeping when you get home. A bad "day's" sleep heading into another night shift is even more miserable and potentially is dangerous. Provigil®

116

(modafinil) and Nuvigil® (amrodafinil) are new medications that promote "wakefulness." They are similar to amphetamines, but don't have the abuse potential. They are very effective at maintaining performance levels despite night shifts and sleep deprivation. As opposed to caffeine (which only requires a Starbucks card), these medicines do require a doctor's prescription and should be used under supervision. But, if you are really struggling and don't have other employment options, a prescription may be your best bet. **(Sack)**

Shift Work Disorder: Five Tips for Maintaining: Productivity and Health

1. Take a short nap right before work.
2. If possible, get bright light at the <u>beginning</u> of your shift.
3. On your way home, avoid exposure to bright light so you can sleep when you get there. Dark goggles are hot!
4. Take Melatonin on the way to bed and sleep in a very dark room in the morning.
5. Caffeine early in the shift improves alertness. Provigil® (modafinil) or Nuvigil® (armodafinil) taken early in the shift to help maintain wakefulness. Do not to use either caffeine or a stimulant too late in the shift. They will prevent sleeping when you finally have the chance.

Section 5: Odd Sleep Behaviors

"Fasten your seatbelts. It's going to be a bumpy night."
Joseph Mankiewicz

     Weird things sometimes happen during sleep. Most of these are categorized as Parasomnias. The term is broken down like this: Para- (around or with) and -somnia (sleep). These are behaviors and activities that occur without conscious control during slumber. And if you are physically busy when you are supposed to be resting and restoring, you will probably wake up tired.

     Parasomnias are triggered by a variety of things; caffeine, stress, illness, chronic sleep deprivation, head injuries, psychiatric illness, and medication/drug use among others. So having a complete medical history is important to diagnosis.

     Most of the time family members are the ones who rat you out. If you sleep alone, and no one is there to witness your carousing, the only clue may be unexplainable daytime sleepiness, or a broken lamp. On occasion a sleep study is needed to document what and when you do at night.

     There are five major types: Arousal, Movement, Hallucination, REM Sleep associated, and Bedwetting. We will explore each in the chapters that follow. It may well be a strange ride. Buckle up.

Chapter 8: The Arousal Parasomnias or "Things That Go Weird in the Night."

Confusional Arousals

Q. My wife says that I awaken in the night, sitting up in bed looking dazed and confused. Then I roll over and go back to sleep. I never remember any of this. What is going on?

You are having Confusional Arousals (or Sleep Drunkenness). These are the simplest of the parasomnias and the easiest to diagnose. During deep (Stage 3) sleep, often in the first half of the night, you seemingly awaken and act confused, and then go happily back to sleep no worse for the wear. Most of the time a Confusional Arousal is no big deal. If these occur frequently and disrupt your wife's sleep, she may disagree. Medication effects and sleep deprivation are the most common causes. Confusional Arousals are not considered signs of any more worrisome sleep problems.

There is no treatment. Make sure you are sleeping enough. Review any medications you started prior to these episodes. And finally, reassure your wife that you will be okay.

Q. My wife is scaring the daylights out of me. She wakes up hollering and freaked out. I freak out and try to settle her down but she doesn't seem to even notice that I'm there. Then it's over and she goes back to sleep. In the morning she swears nothing happened the night before. What is _that_ all about!?!

She is experiencing Night Terrors. More accurately she is having them but you are the one experiencing them. Night Terrors are really scary for the bed partner. Seemingly out of nowhere, she sits up screaming, sweating, and acting as if Bigfoot is chasing her through the Canadian wilderness! Even though she seems wide awake she won't respond to you. And if you try to calm her she may resist forcefully and even push you away. Then she lies down like nothing ever happened and goes peacefully back to sleep. You are probably not sleeping again so quickly, though. In the morning over coffee the conversation usually goes something like this. "What happened to you last night? You scared me to death!" "I slept like a baby. I have no idea what you are talking about."

Night Terrors usually occur in the first half of the night and are not associated with dreams and REM sleep. They are also rare in adults. Instigating factors in susceptible people include stress, illness, caffeine, and/or sleep deficiency (maybe due to other sleep diagnoses). The terrors often go away when she catches up on her sleep. If not, or if she is becoming increasingly violent and you worry she may hurt herself (or you), sedatives (like Klonopin® (clonazepam) are useful. If treatment isn't helping, it is time for a sleep study to see what else is going on.

Sleep Walking

Q. My family says I am wandering around upstairs late at night. I don't believe them. Am I crazy or are they?

You have Somnambulism - Somn- (sleep) and -ambulism (ambulating/walking). Sleep walking adults often did so as kids, though most people outgrow it by age 8. Contrary to common belief, "walking" in your sleep does not necessarily mean strolling around the house. Just sitting up in bed counts. If your family awakens you during your nighttime journey you will be very confused, like a Confusional Arousal. As usual, there is no morning recall of your expedition.

Obviously there are some safety issues that accompany Sleep Walking. Falling down stairs (asleep or awake) is never a good thing. Providing a safe sleep environment is really important for injury prevention.

Like a lot of Parasomnias, insufficient sleep and stress can precipitate Sleep Walking. If a good night's sleep isn't the antidote, it is possible to treat with medication. Sedatives are effective, particularly if the Sleep Walking is disruptive to your spouse or your safety is at risk.

Sleep Talking

Q. Fortunately, he hasn't said anything that has made me mad at him yet, but my boyfriend is waking me up every night with his talking. Help!

Sleep talking or Somniloquy (Somn- (sleep) plus -iloquy (talking)) is very common. Most often it happens in non-REM sleep or during brief awakenings and readjustments that we have from time to time at night. Nonsense usually comes out, though the sleep talker can be disturbingly lucid at times. (Once, while sharing a room on vacation, my son sat up in bed and announced to all who would listen: "It is a series of 7 books, the first of which is the smallest.") Like the other Parasomnias, your boyfriend will not have any recall of what was said. Sleep Talking is of no consequence to the orator. Sharing a sleeping space is difficult with all the chatter though. If he is disruptive to your good night's sleep, a sedative can be prescribed – for him.

THE CRAZY STUFF

Q. I've heard of people doing very bizarre stuff during sleep– is it really true?

Yes, there are such things as Sleep Eating, Sleep Sex (Sexomnia), and Sleep Violence. Unfortunately, these problems do exist. They are odd and interesting to read about. But these Parasomnias are disruptive at best and tragic at worst. I will touch upon each to inform and entertain you.

Sleep Related Eating Disorder (SRED)

Taking a stroll to the refrigerator and eating a nighttime snack may not be that unusual. It takes a turn toward the bizarre if someone seems sound asleep when it happens. This type of behavior may indicate a psychiatric condition or a bizarre seizure disorder. But sometimes it is a Parasomnia.

We call this one "Sleep Related Eating Disorder" (SRED). "Sleeping" people who suffer from SRED go to the kitchen, or

121

wherever else one might find food (more on that later), and eat. What do they eat? Well, just about anything. Consuming buttered cigarettes is the craziest "food" item I have heard about. Consider this a Confusional Arousal with the Munchies. People with SRED usually (80%) have other sleep disorders like Sleep Walking, Restless Leg Syndrome, and/or Periodic Limb Movements. Some have Obstructive Sleep Apnea as well. Clearly a sleep issue is going on here. **(Auger)** Anti-depressants, sedatives, and anti-psychotics have all been implicated in causing SRED. As you might guess from that list of medications, psychiatric disease often goes hand in hand with SRED.

Sleep Related Eating is often a very aggressive and uncoordinated activity that occasionally leads to injury. Some people eat so ravenously they wake up with bruises. If someone is awakened on the way to the refrigerator they won't confess to hunger or any desire to eat. Interestingly, alcohol is never on the menu, even for alcoholics.

Because there are probably numerous causes for SRED, there are many different medications used for therapy. If there are no other sleep or medical disorders, an anti-epilepsy medication called Topamax® (topiramate)is the most effective medication. Sleep aids (like Klonopin® (clonazepam) antidepressant medications (like Prozac® (fluoxetine), Paxil® (paroxetine), Obsessive Compulsive Disorder treatments, (Luvox® (fluvoxamine)), and even codeine are also potentially helpful. Successful treatment is very satisfying. In one study, participants lost up to 20 pounds when their SRED was treated with medication. **(Auger)**

Psychiatric Night Eating Problems

Other nighttime eaters consciously make this choice. Some morbidly obese people have Night Eating Syndrome (NES). People with NES decide while fully awake to consume up to 25% of their caloric intake after they have gone to bed. Binge Eaters and Bulimics often feel compelled to eat at night. Most people with Night Eating Syndrome need psychiatric help. **(Schenck)** This is not a Parasomnia.

Klein Levin Syndrome

Klein Levin Syndrome (KLS) affects adolescent males. These young men eat and sleep excessively most likely due to a brain dysfunction. A more complete discussion is found in Chapter 13, Narcolepsy and the Hypersomnias. (NIH)

Q. How do I know if I have Sleep Related Eating Disorder versus these other eating disorders?

If there is suspicion that this really is a Parasomnia, see your friendly neighborhood Sleep Medicine doctor. A sleep study is in order too, though not with the usual protocol. The array of monitors is the same. But video observation is critical. To make sure you have a chance to misbehave, food is left in the room some distance away from the bed. If you get up to eat, the sleep technician goes into the room to interact with you. If you really have Sleep Related Eating Disorder you will be arousable and confused and baffled when the tech checks in with you. Also, you will be "awake" based on brain waves measured for the sleep study. In contrast, a person with a psychiatric disorder will be fully cognizant of their actions and might even be defensive, having been disrupted in the middle of a snack.

Sleep Sex (Sexomnia)

Some people become sexually active while asleep. Yes, this really occurs and can be a problem, as strange as that may sound. It occurs in non-REM sleep, like most all of the Parasomnias. Studied in the sleep lab, the body responds exactly like any other intimate and sexually stimulating situation. Orgasms even happen! Sexomnia patients occasionally report the sex as if it happened during a dream. The sleeping performer rarely lights up a cigarette and engages in pillow talk afterward, though. In fact, upon awakening in the morning, there is usually no recollection of the busy night. Loud moaning, dirty language, and aggressive masturbation occur. Actual oral, anal and vaginal sex may happen, too. If the person chosen to be the object of your "affections" is so inclined to participate it might not be such a bad thing. But if the Sexomniac happens upon

123

someone who has not consented to such behavior, trouble may ensue. And it is especially appalling if the act occurs with a minor.

Sounds like a nighttime law drama plot? "Law and Order, Special Victims Unit" played out this very same scenario. In this particular episode, the boyfriend was the culprit. He started having sexual relations with his girlfriend with whom he shared a bed, apparently in his sleep. The trouble started when he Sleep Walked into her little sister's room, who was not so excited by his presence. Legal quandaries and drama began to brew. The popular doctor show "House" once had a similar story line. Art imitates life. Both truth and fiction can be strange.

Most of the people who really do suffer from sleep-sex have other sleep issues. Most are sleepwalkers and have strong family histories of the same. There are some experts who will argue that sexomnia is an elaborate form of sleep walking with automatic behaviors that just happen to be intimate in nature.

Thirty-five percent of people with Sexomnia have had legal problems because of their behavior. Real life examples of these nighttime shenanigans are common with many descriptions of "Sexomniacs" in the medical and legal literature. For example, a man in England was acquitted of rape when his Parasomnia explained his nighttime sexual behavior. **(Ibrahim)** Some people are more considerate lovers during their Parasomnia-related sex. Others exhibit violent sexual behavior. One woman even claimed that she liked the passion despite the bruises from her otherwise sleeping husband. Self-injury has also happened.

Men, typically in their 20's and 30's, are most likely to have Sexomnia. The diagnosis often brings shame and trouble. The lack of control over such a basic and meaningful part of life can be really disturbing, not to mention the effect this has on the recipients of their attentions. **(Schenck)**

Most Sexomniacs want to have their unwanted conduct fixed. Treatment is usually very successful with the use of a sedative (like Klonopin® (clonazepam). **(Guilleminault)** Hopefully, the recipient of his or her nighttime affection isn't too disappointed.

Sleep Violence

Now we are getting into the real CSI stuff; the dark corner of the sleep world. It is a tragic place for those who really suffer Sleep Violence, both for the person acting out and the person(s) being acted upon. It is also a place for a few perps who try to blame "sleep" for their malicious acts. Sleep related violence is as unusual as it gets.

Sleep Violence may actually be a merging of several parasomnias including Sleep Walking and Night Terrors; the terror being translated into action with sometimes dire results. Just like with Sexomnia, most of the people who have this also have a history of other Parasomnias throughout their lives (e.g. sleep walking, confusional arousals, sleep terrors, and/or nightmares). It occurs in the first part of the night in non-REM sleep just like the other parasomnias.

A typical scenario is this: you are sleep walking, perhaps after a sleep terror or confusional arousal, when confronted with a person or situation to which you react. In this altered mental state of disordered sleep, violence can erupt against someone in the wrong place at the wrong time. The consequences of Sleep Violence are obviously disturbing. **(Pressman)**

Once again, enter Hollywood. Yes, art again imitates life. The Sleepwalker Killing was a made for TV movie in 1997 starring Hilary Swank. In the movie, a man kills his mother-in-law (cue the jokes) and injures his father-in-law. His defense: his actions occurred while he was sleep. No spoiler here. You can check it out if you want to know how it ends. **(IMBD)**

More tragically, and real, are the stories that art is imitating. One popularly reported event occurred in England in 2009. A devoted husband who suffered from sleepwalking and night terrors his entire life strangled his wife to death in her sleep. At home, understanding his propensity to nighttime activity, the couple slept in separate rooms for safety. While on holiday he dreamt that someone was breaking into the camper they shared. When he awoke and realized what he had done he immediately made an emergency call. He was acquitted of all charges. **(Guardian)**

In this case, as in others that are well documented in the legal and popular press, a defendant with a diagnosis of real Sleep

Violence is not held responsible for their behavior and is therefore not culpable. Sleepwalking and violence are legally deemed to be different from insanity, unconsciousness, or automatic behavior. In court it is the responsibility of defense lawyers to establish that the accused was really asleep at the time. **(Boston Law Review)** Complete psychological and psychiatric testing is always done in these cases. Sleep studies and complete sleep histories are necessary if Sleep Violence is the defense. Typically there is a strong personal and family history of sleepwalking and talking and the like. Sleep studies sometimes demonstrate decreased slow wave/deep sleep. Abnormal behavior may even be documented during the study. If the lawyers can get confirmation that the patient has a propensity to parasomnia and has all the right answers on interrogation, they might get a not guilty verdict. If not…

How often this really occurs is anyone's guess. One large-scale telephone survey from Europe came up with a number of 1.7%, which seems high to me. I can just imagine the call…Researcher, yawning, "Have you ever been violent in your sleep?" Random sarcastic European answering the phone, "Uh, yeah, sure. I do that all the time." Suddenly excited researcher, "REALLY? Can you tell me about it…" Not sure about the validity of that data. Most of the people who admitted to Sleep Violence were younger and slightly more likely to be men. Over 30% reported injuring themselves or others during an episode. Triggers of Sleep Violence are the usual suspects: alcohol, excessive Caffeine, illegal drugs, sleep deprivation, stress, and anxiety. **(Ohahon)**

So how do we get this to go away? By treating the any underlying sleep disorder. When the other Parasomnia is fixed, so will the Parasomnia related violence. In the meantime, create a safe environment for you and your family/friends at night. That way you can do whatever you do without injuring yourself or others.

Chapter 9: The Movement Parasomnias (A.K.A. Dancin' the Watusi)

There are a wide variety of Movement Parasomnias: repetitive motions, abnormal sensations, and the gnashing of teeth. These can be really disruptive to you and your bed partner. If you are suffering (in either role) read on...

Limb Movements

Q. Apparently I am kicking when I am asleep, or so my wife says. I keep waking her up. I, on the other hand, am sleeping just fine, thank you very much. But I would like to be invited back to our bed. What can we do about this?

Periodic Limb Movements of Sleep (PLMS) is a rather common related problem. Like a lot of these Parasomnias, the person suffering sleep disruption is your bed partner. The diagnosis is made if you demonstrate characteristic rhythmic and repetitive movements, typically of the legs, at least 5 times an hour during a sleep study. You can't have any other sleep disorder, either. Limb movements are frequently seen during sleep studies for Sleep Apnea. If they persist after the OSA is treated the diagnosis is entertained. PLMS often goes with Restless Legs Syndrome (see below).

When the movements begin to disrupt your sleep they are reclassified into a full-blown medical problem, apologies to the wife. Periodic Limb Movement Disorder (PLMD) means that you have 5+ extremity movements per hour that disrupt your sleep and are associated with daytime sleepiness and impairment.

So we treat PLMS to maintain marital bliss if your bed partner is about to kick you out of bed. We treat PLMD when your sleep is disrupted, too. We use the same sort of medications that treat Parkinson's Disease. Medicines that act like Dopamine in the brain are very effective with low side effects. However, there is some controversy as to whether it is appropriate to expose you to medication for this particular problem. **(Aurora)** I'd say if this is really disrupting YOUR sleep it is worth considering a medication for it.

Q. When I try to go to sleep I feel like there are worms crawling inside my legs. The only relief I get is if I walk around. It is driving me crazy! Am I crazy?

No, you are not insane. It sounds like you are suffering from Restless Legs Syndrome (RLS). This is really miserable problem that is surprisingly common. Estimates say that up to 10% of Americans experience RLS. **(Silber)** Those abnormal sensations can be just about anything: pins and needles (can't it be just pins or needles?), burning, throbbing, aching, electrical shocks, and creepy crawlies. My personal favorite is christened "Elvis Legs" – the intense need to move the lower extremities. Timing is the biggest problem with RLS. These feelings usually kick up at night when you are starting to settle down to sleep. Moving around helps to relieve the discomfort. In the extreme case, Restless Legs Syndrome can become so intense and unrelenting that relaxation is almost impossible. It is hard to sleep when you feel a need to get up and walk around to quiet the snakes in your legs. Also people with RLS have a lot of limb movement after they go to sleep. See the previous section for a more in depth discussion of Periodic Limb Movement Disorder (PLMD).

The diagnosis of Restless Legs Syndrome requires all four of the following criteria:
1. The symptoms occur mostly at night and are gone in the morning
2. There is an overwhelming desire to move to relieve the symptoms. There are often feelings of numbness or pain in the legs as well.
3. The whole thing is triggered by relaxation and an attempt to sleep.
4. The weird feelings are relieved by movement and stay away as long as you keep moving.

We don't yet understand the cause of RLS. Iron deficiency is sometimes blamed. Decreased iron may decrease Dopamine (a brain chemical) levels. Low Dopamine levels may be the ultimate cause of RLS. Your doctor should check your iron levels, iron binding capacity, and ferritin levels with a blood test. If these are low, taking supplemental iron is necessary and may be curative. **(Brindani)**

128

If improving your iron stores doesn't work, there are effective treatments with medications that act like dopamine in the brain. The newer drugs (Requip® (ropinirole) and Mirapex®)) have low side effects. They don't tend to cause "augmentation" (a worsening of the symptoms because of the medications) or stomach upset like the previous generation of drugs. Like with any medication there are down sides, including reports of unusual behaviors and problems with impulse control: hypersexuality, impulsive gambling, excessive eating, and compulsive shopping. Fortunately these effects are rare and stop when the medication is stopped.

Alternative treatments for Restless Legs Syndrome are available if you are not responding to the standard approaches. The pain medication codeine, for some reason, seems to be effective. It is well tolerated with few side effects. Parkinson's medications that increase the levels of Dopamine in the brain are also effective though they have a much higher rate of side effects. They are also more likely to amplify the intensity of the RLS (augmentation). **(Aurora)** Also, the anticonvulsant medications Neurontin® (gabapentin) and Lyrica® (pregabalin) have been shown to have excellent effect without the risk of augmentation. **(Buchfurher)**

Q. Frequently when I am trying to fall asleep I jump. My arm or leg shoots out and scares my partner and me awake. What's going on?

These common and normal occurrences are called Sleep Starts, or Hypnic Jerks. These sudden, involuntary muscle contractions occur just as you are falling asleep. They are completely benign and raise no health concerns. Like most Parasomnias, Sleep Starts are brought about by fatigue, insufficient sleep, and stress.

Sensory Sleep Starts also occur. Instead of a sudden movement, you might have a sudden odd feeling in a limb that intrudes just as you are falling asleep. These are also of no concern.

Teeth Grinding

Q. My husband is making such a racket at night. His teeth grinding is so loud it is disrupting my sleep. What is he doing and why? Fix him!

He is bruxing. Really, that is what it is called. Bruxism, or teeth grinding/clenching is extremely common. Kids do it all the time. Up to 3% of adults grind their teeth. Why people do it is a mystery. Physical and/or mental stress may induce Bruxism in adults. So de-stressing is helpful. Most of the time, though, Bruxism occurs with no obvious reason. It is not without consequences, though.

If the bed partner doesn't protest, the grinder often will. TMJ (temporomandibular, or jaw, joint) problems are common complaints of chronic Bruxers. Headaches, jaw pain, ear pain, and tooth wear result from the stress and strain on the teeth, joint, and chewing muscles. Cracked teeth may require reparative dental work.

There is no known treatment besides prevention of dental injury. Mouthpieces (over-the-counter or custom-made by your dentist) provide a cushion between the teeth and take pressure off the jaw joints. Tooth-guards also quiet the noise of the enamel being chipped off, helping your bed partner sleep. Find relief from jaw or ear pain by staying away from chewy foods, taking anti-inflammatory medications (like ibuprofen or naproxen) and applying heat.

Chapter 10: The Hallucination Parasomnias (A.K.A. "What the...?")

Hallucination is defined as the mistaken perception of something seen, heard, felt, tasted, or even smelled, accompanied by a compelling sense of reality. Psychotic people are the classic example, having conversations with unseen voices or seeing things that aren't there. On occasion, hallucinations occur during the sleep of otherwise normal people. They are also associated with Narcolepsy. So we take your complaints seriously if hallucinating is a regular part of your night.

Hypnopompic/Hypnogogic Hallucinations

Q. I am having the weirdest visions when I am falling asleep. I swear I saw my Uncle Ernie fly-fishing over the bed! Am I going crazy?

No. You aren't losing your mind. You have experienced a hypnogogic (upon going to sleep) or hypnopompic (upon awakening) hallucination. While they are unsettling and unnerving, sleep hallucinations are not worrisome. Nor do they mean that you are losing your mind or that Uncle Ernie is secretly fly-fishing over the top of your bed. It is an odd experience but nothing more. Often these hallucinations are coupled with a sleep paralysis episode, which makes a creepy hallucination that much scarier.

Sleep hallucinations are more common than you might think. In one study 29% of college students reported experiencing sleep paralysis and most of them had hallucinated as well. **(Cheyne)** This phenomenon is well described through the ages. In fact, in 1664 a Dutch physician published a collection of his patient's experiences called "The devil lay upon her and held her down." **(Kompahje)** We think that most of these unnerving but otherwise unconcerning events occur at the border between awake and asleep, which is why they are associated with Narcolepsy (see Chapter 13.)

Exploding Head Syndrome

Q. I think my house exploded today, but nothing was blown up. I heard a HUGE NOISE just as I was waking up. Scared me to

death. But when I went to look what happened, there nothing wrong. I really am going crazy now, right?

You have experienced one of my very favorite diagnoses: Exploding Head Syndrome. A loud sound, bright flash of light, or even a painful feeling is experienced quite suddenly as you are falling asleep or waking up. Needless to say, it is quite the disturbing experience. Sleep brainwave studies reveal that these events occur as you are transitioning into or out of sleep. **(Sachs)** While having an "Exploding Head" is frightening, it isn't dangerous. There are no known medical problems that result from or occur because of the "head explosions," unless you count being afraid to go to sleep. Sleep anxiety is common if you have these regularly.

Treatment is usually reassurance by a sleep specialist that there in fact is no detonation going on and the world is not exploding. With time this problem usually resolves. Healthy sleep habits are most often curative. If that doesn't work we can always try some medication. Toprax® (topiramate), an anti-epileptic used for migraine headaches and Anafranil® (clomipramine), a tricyclic antidepressant, have both been used successfully.

Chapter 11: REM Associated Parasomnias

All of the Parasomnias thus far described occur in non-REM sleep, meaning non-dream sleep. The REM sleep stage is where dreams occur. If you need a review on REM and non-REM sleep please go to Chapter 1, What is Sleep?, for a refresher course.

REM is very different from the other stages of sleep. Normally, the brain physically inhibits movement during dream sleep. Upsetting this balance has consequences. Movement issues during REM sleep can become unintended adventures. Too little movement can be terrifying. And if we experience REM too vividly sleep can get a little scary. Read on…

Nightmare Disorder

Q. I have started having really bad dreams. I awaken at 3 or 4 in the morning, sweating and shaking, scared out of my wits because of these crazy visions I am having. What is going on?

You are having nightmares. The question is why and what can be done about them?

Because REM sleep is when most dreams happen, and because REM sleep is mostly in the early morning hours, nightmares usually occur after midnight. Nightmare Disorder afflicts 4% or fewer adults. Almost 80% of people with Nightmare Disorder suffer from Post-Traumatic Stress Disorder (PTSD) (e.g. veterans, abuse and trauma victims). Life stressors and/or lack of sleep often precipitate bad dreams.

Some medications are known to produce bad dreams also. Inderal® (propranolol), a beta blocker-high blood pressure drug, is known as the "nightmare drug" because it increases the REM stage sleep and dreaming.

To garner a diagnosis of Nightmare Disorder, your bad dreams must be disruptive to sleep and daily life. Some people are really taken over by the nightmares and begin to have "sleep anxiety." They are apprehensive just thinking about sleeping and returning to their horrifying dreams. Effective treatments exist with and without medication.

Image Rehearsal Therapy (IRT) has a good track record. With this method you consciously redirect the dream to your liking. The procedure goes like this. When you wake up after a nightmare you write it down. During the light of day, you decide how to flip the script. You edit the dream to change the subject matter, plot, or finale, to make it positive. This exercise is repeated 10-20 minutes daily until you extinguish your fear and redirect you dream.

Systematic Desensitization is another approach usually taken under the guidance of a counselor. This technique aims to take the fear out of your particular nightmare. Gradually, and increasingly, the subject is talked about, confronted, and finally, stared down. You steadily and progressively dismiss your fear during the day. When it doesn't scare you anymore, the nightmare has no further power over you.

Progressive Deep Muscle Relaxation practices show promise as well. Reducing physical stress allows you to release tension and anxiety before you head off to sleep. You start by contracting and then relaxing your face, then your neck, arms, chest, stomach, thighs, calves, and finally your feet, one part of the body at a time. This helps to relieve the bodily tightness that accompanies mental apprehension as you go to sleep. Less trepidation equals less worry and fewer nightmares.

Several medications are available that act specifically to help prevent nightmares. One blood pressure medication (Minipress® (prazosin)) inhibits one of the adrenalin receptors (α_1) in the brain, reducing much of the nightmare and your reaction to it. Another (Catapress® (clonidine)) actually stimulates another of the adrenalin receptors (α_2) to give the same effect. Go figure. Both are particularly effective for people who also suffer from PTSD. **(Aurora)**

Sedation is a possibility too. Knocking you out for a while may help you get through the stressors and anxiety that are perpetuating the nightmares. Some of the anti-anxiety/anti-depressant medications like SSRIs (selective serotonin reuptake inhibitors like Prozac® (fluoxetine) and antidepressants (like Elavil® (amitriptyline)) can decrease the amount of REM sleep you get. Most of the time this is a negative, contributing to daytime sleepiness. For you it might help to decrease REM, where your Nightmare Disorder occurs.

134

REM Behavior Disorder: (A.K.A. Help! Save me from the giant purple alligator!)

Q. My Uncle Fred relives fighting in Korea in his sleep. What in the heck is he doing? He might hurt Aunt Mertyl!

Uncle Fred most likely has REM Behavior Disorder (RBD). Consider REM Behavior Disorder a nightmare in action.

Usually, when you hit REM sleep your brain shuts down your ability to move. That way you are protected from reacting to a crazy dream sequence. RDB disables the muscle shut-off switch. So, if a giant purple alligator, or a North Korean soldier, is trying to kill you in the dream you naturally try to protect yourself, reacting physically and sometimes aggressively in your sleep. This behavior is potentially dangerous to you or those around you.

Only about .05% of the population has REM Behavior Disorder. Over 80% are men who started having symptoms in their late 50's. A substantial minority of people with RBD also have, or will develop, Parkinson's Disease and/or some form of Dementia. **(Trotti)** Rarely, anti-depressant/anti-anxiety medications are linked to the onset of RBD. **(Kierlin)**

REM Behavior Disorder is diagnosed in the sleep lab. Normally, the muscles on the chin and the front of the leg we monitor during the study have very little activity during REM sleep. This is one of the cardinal signs of stage REM. Someone with RBD exhibits normal muscle tone during stage REM. Combine this sleep study finding with behavior reported by the family (and potentially observed during the study) and the diagnosis is made.

Treatment is very simple. Klonopin® (clonazepam) is effective in 90% of people with RDB. If you can't take Klonopin®, Melatonin is effective in 70-80% of the time.

Sleep Paralysis

Q. I woke up this morning and couldn't move. I was completely aware of being awake but was completely immobile for what seemed like forever. Finally I was able to get out of bed. What happened? Did I have a stroke or something?

135

You probably awoke in a REM sleep stage during which you were physically unable to move. For that short period of time before the muscles were released to normal activity you experienced Sleep Paralysis. It is a remarkably common occurrence. In the US almost 8% of the general population has had an episode. It is reported more frequently in students. Over 30% of people with psychiatric problems have experienced Sleep Paralysis. **(Sharpless)** Fun fact: up to 40% of the population in Japan reports having had this experience. **(Fukuda)**

In a perfectly normal person who has otherwise normal sleep an episode like this is of no great concern. It may be scary, but it doesn't mean anything else. It is brief (though it may not feel short to you) and harmless (though at the time it is frightening) and does not indicate any other medical problem.

These episodes are usually caused by a lack of sleep. If you are snoozing enough and are still frequently having Sleep Paralysis, see your doctor. Recurrent episodes associated with daytime sleepiness indicate the possibility of Narcolepsy (see Chapter 13.).

Chapter 12: Bedwetting (Enuresis)

Bedwetting (in medicalese – Nocturnal Enuresis) is a taboo subject, especially for adults. It happens though. And if you are suffering from Enuresis, you should know that there is help. Forget the feelings of shame and humiliation. This is a medical bladder control problem, not a character flaw or sign of physical weakness.

Q. I am mortified to tell you this but I still wet the bed as an adult. I wear adult diapers to bed, but want to stop. What can I do about this embarrassing problem?

Enuresis in adults is usually an extension of childhood bedwetting. It occurs because you do not arouse from sleep in response to the urge to go to pee. This problem tends to run in families. It may be a big family secret. Don't let it stay that way. Get your problem fixed with the help of your doctor. There are lots of successful approaches.

First, exercise to help strengthen your control muscles and increase bladder capacity. To increase bladder volume and your ability to control and regulate your pee, practice holding your urine longer and longer while you are awake. Kegel exercises strengthen bladder and pelvic muscles. These are accomplished by squeezing your pelvic muscles as if you are repeatedly stopping your urine in midstream. Stronger muscles mean better control.

You also need to prepare yourself at night. Limit fluid intake several hours before bedtime. Urinate right before you go to bed. Occasionally it is useful to plan an awakening to urinate halfway through the night. Set your beside alarm clock for 2:00AM to go to the toilet. Even if you don't feel an urge to go, you will empty your bladder and have a better chance of staying dry the rest of the night.

Bed alarms that sense wetness are available. The alarm is triggered if you start to pee. Hopefully with time you will begin to recognize the urge and awaken on your own.

There is not much research on adult Enuresis. Most of the recommendations are extensions from pediatric studies. However, there are helpful medications. The antidepressant Tofranil® (imipramine) may help, but its use is controversial. Drugs that decrease urine production are also available. A nasal spray, called DDAVP® (desmopressin), limits kidney production for several hours after use. Taking it at bedtime, especially when combined with fluid restriction, may be helpful.

If your bladder is overactive, medications that relax those muscles may help. Detrol® (tolterodine) or Ditropan® (oxybutynin) are commonly prescribed. They work by blocking the nerve stimulus that initiates bladder contraction and peeing.

Finally, as you said, wearing an adult diaper to bed protects the sheets. They are very effective but at best are socially awkward, as you probably already know. **(NAFC)**

If you have Obstructive Sleep Apnea, the picture may be brighter. Normally, Apnea and peeing go hand in hand. Numerous awakenings that occur with apneas bring awareness to your bladder situation. Thus you get up to pee. If your Sleep Apnea is extreme, you may be in heart failure. The fluid that collected in your lungs and legs during the day goes back into circulation when you lie down to sleep. Urine production goes up causing frequent awakenings to pee. Even worse, if you can't awaken fully due to the severity of your Sleep Apnea, you may wet the bed. The good news here is that if Obstructive Sleep Apnea is treated, excessive urine production and bedwetting improve. **(Kramer)**

Lastly, anyone with new onset bedwetting needs to be evaluated for some form of urological problems. Bladder dysfunction, incontinence, and other plumbing problems are correctable causes of enuresis. **(Whiteside)**

Section 6: Excessive Sleepiness

"I think I'm a narcoleptic. I could sleep on a railway track with a train running over me, in-between the rails."
Dan Aykroyd

Chapter 13: Narcolepsy and the Hypersomnias (Dig that funky sound...)

Very simply put, Hyper- (really a huge amount) and – Somnia (drowsiness) add up to being incredibly sleepy. The question is, why are you so tired? If the sleepiness is a disruptive problem to your life, and isn't caused by other medical problems, medications, or another sleep diagnosis, it is time to see your friendly local sleep specialist to figure out how to get back in the game.

Narcolepsy

Q. I am tired all of the time. I also have a lot of weird things happening to me day and night. Do I have Narcolepsy?

Maybe. Understanding Narcolepsy requires some knowledge of sleep and sleep stages (learn more in Chapter 1, What is Sleep?). Quick review: Stages 1, 2 and 3 describe progressively deeper sleep stages. REM (Rapid Eye Movement) sleep is the "deepest" stage and where most dreams occur. During REM, movement is inhibited, protecting you from acting out your dreams.

Narcolepsy is poorly regulated and disorganized sleep. Because sleep and wake is so chaotically controlled, they can occur at any time; middle of the day, middle of the night, it doesn't seem to matter. Constant drowsiness results from slipping in and out of sleep without a schedule. The diagnosis is typically made in the late teens and early twenties when symptoms are increasingly upsetting to daytime function.

Cataplexy is the term that describes more severe and intrusive symptoms that occur in a small percentage of people with Narcolepsy. Falling suddenly, feeling weak limbed, or slack jawed, often when expressing intense emotions (laughter, tears, or fright) is typical. These symptoms are thought to be the sudden intrusion of a REM sleep cycle that inhibits muscle tone during wakefulness. Why these events are triggered by emotion is not clear. Spontaneously slipping into a brief REM sleep at the end of a hilarious joke is embarrassing at very least.

Visual and auditory hallucinations when falling asleep (hypnogogic hallucinations) or when awakening (hypnopompic hallucinations) are also common. These can be very disturbing until you know why you are having them.

Severe daytime sleepiness makes just getting through the day a real chore. Depression is common and frequently needs to be addressed. Also, weight gain and obesity are common in people with Narcolepsy.

If all of this sounds familiar a presumptive diagnosis of Narcolepsy, with or without Cataplexy, is entertained. Because the treatments are such a big deal, confirmation of the diagnosis with a sleep study or two is necessary. You may need genetic testing also.

Q. How do you make the diagnosis of Narcolepsy?

The evaluation usually begins in your primary care doctor's office. If you complain of way-overboard sleepiness, he or she will rule out all of the usual suspects (anemia, thyroid problems, viral illnesses, hepatitis, etc.). If all of those are negative, you should be referred to your local sleep medicine doc. At that visit the focus is solely on sleep.

General mental and physical health details that relate to sleep are explored. It is crucial to be completely honest with your sleep specialist. Drugs (legal and otherwise) and alcohol have real impacts on your sleep. (See Chapter 17 for a more complete discussion on Medications and Sleep) There is no judgment during a doctor's visit. All information is completely confidential. You will also be questioned about snoring, apnea, sleep behaviors, sleep timing, family sleep problems, and cataplexy symptoms.

You will fill out an Epworth Sleepiness Scale, a questionnaire (referenced in Chapter 3, Insomnia and Chapter 5, Sleep Apnea) to measure how you describe your own sleepiness. Depression, anxiety, and other mental health issues are discussed. All of this information is coupled with your physical examination, to get an idea about whether Narcolepsy is even on the list. If so, we give you an assignment on the way to the sleep studies (yes there are two – keep reading.)

Your homework consists of filling out a Sleep Log for the two weeks prior to your sleep studies. The Sleep Log (on the next page for your viewing pleasure) is an often-revealing look at your sleep patterns. During this period you write down your best estimate of when you get into bed, go to sleep, wake up and get out of bed. That includes waking in the middle of the night to go to the bathroom, naps during the day, and your normal bed and wake up times. The hours and pattern of your sleep is graphically displayed on the chart. If you have the typically disordered sleep characteristic of Narcolepsy, it helps make case for the diagnosis. If it demonstrates sleep patterns consistent with completely different sleep issues (e.g. Circadian Rhythm Disorder, Insomnia, severe sleep deprivation etc.) we switch gears and reassess.

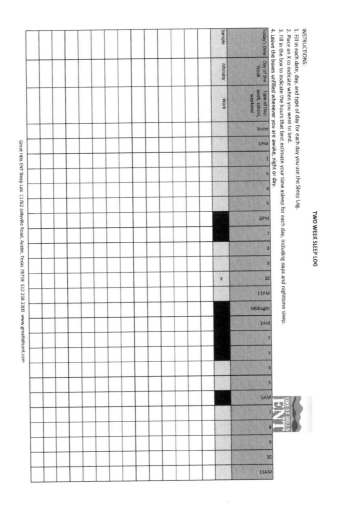

If no other sleep finding is obvious, a run of the mill diagnostic sleep study is your next step. First, it is really important to measure sleep and stages. Second, ruling out Sleep Apnea or other diagnoses is imperative. If you have another sleep disorder it needs to be treated before Narcolepsy is considered. And finally, you need to sleep as well as you can the night before the second study. Sleep deprivation renders the very specific Narcolepsy study inaccurate.

143

If the overnight sleep is not indicative of any other sleep diagnosis, and you have had at least 6 hours of sleep, we proceed with the second part of our inquiry.

Honestly, the last thing you want after a diagnostic sleep study is to stay hooked up to the monitors and continue testing the rest of the next day. But that is exactly what comes next. In the morning a series of additional sleep measurements are taken. This is called the Multiple Sleep Latency Test (MSLT).

It goes like this. After breakfast, you get to freshen up and change into your street clothes. One and a half to 3 hours after you wake up, the next phase begins. Back to bed you go for a nap. Yes, a nap. You lie down in a dark and quiet sleep lab room, dressed and fully monitored. If you fall asleep you get 15 minutes to snooze before you are awakened. If you don't fall asleep after 20 minutes the nap opportunity is over and on go the lights. Over the course of the day you have total of 5 nap opportunities spaced 2 hours apart.

During an MSLT, a normal person with normal rest and alertness takes more than 10 minutes to fall asleep, if they do at all. Sleep deprived people obviously fall asleep more quickly. If you have pathologic sleepiness, like in Narcolepsy, through the course of the day you nod off on average in less than 8 minutes. But that alone isn't enough to make the diagnosis. Going directly into REM sleep at least twice during a minimum of four naps makes the diagnosis of Narcolepsy extremely likely. (We can also count how quickly you got into REM during the sleep study the night before. If you have a REM period that starts immediately after your sleep study starts, you already have one strike against you.)

Just like the rattle in your car that never happens when you drop it off at the mechanic, sleep studies don't always find the diagnosis. Inexplicably you might have a better night's sleep than usual. Or you happen to be more alert because of the lab environment. Despite a negative test, if suspicion remains high, more diagnostic sleep testing (including a repeat MSLT) may be needed until the diagnosis is either solidly ruled in or out.

Q. What other tests that can diagnose Narcolepsy?

Genetic markers (HLA D15 and HLA DQB1*0602) are found in some people with Narcolepsy. DQB1*0602 is more commonly associated with Narcolepsy <u>and</u> Cataplexy. A simple blood test can determine your genetic situation. Orexin, also called hypocretin, is a brain neurotransmitter that is involved in the regulation and maintenance of wakefulness. (Try heading to Chaper 20, The Science of Sleep, if you want more information about brain function and sleep.) It is deficient in many people with Narcolepsy. Finding low orexin levels in spinal fluid also supports the diagnosis. Combined with a positive MSLT and all of your struggles, these other tests confirm the diagnosis and open the door to treatment.

Q. How do you treat Narcolepsy?

As of this writing, there is no therapy that directly treats the brain chemistry causes of Narcolepsy. Treatment focuses on controlling your extreme sleepiness. The medications try to keep you awake during the day and consolidate your sleep at night.

First we keep you awake using stimulants to promote wakefulness during daylight hours. Ritalin® (methylphenidate), Dexedrine® (dextroamphetamine), and Adderall® (amphetamine-dextroamphetamine) are common choices. These medications may sound familiar. They are frequently used to treat Attention Deficit Disorder. They are all related in some way to methamphetamine, so abuse is the biggest potential problem with them. You have to be careful. But, used correctly they are very safe and effective.

Stimulant treatment without the risk of abuse is also available. Provigil® (modafinil) and NuVigil® (armodafinil) maintain wakefulness without the same level of brain "stimulation" as the amphetamines. So the potential for misuse is much less. **(Wise)** These medications are preferred because they are really safe and effective.

Another very simple non-pharmaceutical therapy is napping. If a normal sleeper takes a daytime nap they may have trouble falling asleep at night. For a person with Narcolepsy, planned naps prior to work or class schedules may refresh the mind and promote wakefulness, albeit temporarily.

After keeping you awake during the day, we force you to sleep at night. Xyrem® (sodium oxybate) is our best, and <u>only</u>, option for this part of the equation at this point in time. It knocks you out FAST! You should take the first dose within 15 minutes of when you plan on being asleep, ideally AFTER you get into bed. The next dose is taken two and a half to four hours later, in the middle of the night. **(Black)** Yes, you have to wake up in the middle of the night to take a medicine to stay asleep. The effect of Xyrem® (sodium oxybate) is so short that twice-nightly dosage is needed to achieve the desired effect: consolidated sleep. Sounds odd, but it really works.

There is the no potential for addiction with Xyrem® (sodium oxybate), but it can be abused. It's downside of is somewhat notorious. Xyrem® (sodium oxybate) is a cousin of the notorious "date rape" drug rohypnol. They work the same way. So you have to keep tight control on who has your medication. You also need to be judicious about where you sleep when taking the medication. Because of this misuse potential, Xyrem® (sodium oxybate) is carefully prescribed and supervised in practice. Jazz Pharmaceuticals is the only provider. They have a great patient program that monitors use and helps patients be safe.

Xyrem® (sodium oxybate) has a real impact decreasing daytime sleepiness. And it is the absolute best therapy for reducing Cataplexy symptoms.

Another approach to control Cataplexy is the use of an antidepressant, Effexor® (venlafaxine). **(Mignot)** It is less effective than Xyrem®, but does help treat Depression that frequently accompanies Narcolepsy.

If we can keep you awake and alert during the day and asleep at night, you will be more functional, happier, and productive.

Kleine Levin Syndrome

Q. My teenage son is acting bizarrely, sleeping all of the time, eating when he is not asleep, and acting very inappropriately. We are VERY worried. What is going on?

Kleine Levin Syndrome (KLS) is an extremely rare, episodic form of hypersomnia. It almost, but not exclusively, occurs in adolescent males. A virus is likely the culprit. Most of the time a "flu-like" illness precedes the onset of KLS. Affected kids have extreme sleepiness; snoozing up to 20 hours a day is common. Behavioral problems (excessive eating, irritability, childishness, confusion, hypersexuality, and even hallucinations) also occur and are very disruptive. The episodes last days to weeks and are recurrent for 8-12 years.

Clearly there is some brain dysfunction that is causing your son's disinhibited and somnolent conduct. Because the exact cause is not yet defined, direct treatment is not available. Awake and asleep brain wave patterns are abnormal when he is symptomatic. These normalize when the symptoms wane. **(Ramburg)** We can try to treat the sleepiness with stimulants, but risk increasing his irritability. Mood modulators like Lithobid® (lithium) and Tegretol® (carbempazepine) are additional alternatives. **(NIND)**

While this may sound like a typical teenage boy's behavior, it is MUCH worse. Kleine-Levin is very disruptive to the decade or so that your son may be affected. The only positive is that eventually the problems decrease or disappear altogether.

Idiopathic Hypersomnia

Q. I think my brother has Hypersomnia, or at least he looks tired all of the time. And he sleeps all the time. What gives?

Some people are super tired all of the time for no obvious reason, even if they regularly sleep for a long time. Your brother will likely have all kinds of workup including sleep studies and blood tests. If everything looks normal, he may have Idiopathic (we can't figure out why) Hypersomnia (sleepy all the time). Treatment with stimulants can keep him awake during the day. Provigil® (modafinil), Nuvigil® (armodafinil) and the ADD (Adderall® (amphetamine-dextroamphetamine), Concerta® (methylphenidate), Dexedrine® (dextroamphetamine)) medications are the therapies of choice.

Section 7: Sleep, the Body, and the Mind

"Sleep is that golden chain that ties health and our bodies together."
Thomas Dekker

Chapter 14: Medical Problems and Sleep

Medical problems disrupt all parts of your life, including sleep. And a lack of sleep makes all of your health problems worse. This reciprocal relationship sets up a vicious cycle that negatively impacts both. Managing your health problems, and acknowledging the role that sleep plays in your health, makes a difference.

Pain

Q. I have chronic back/hip/shoulder/neck/you-name-it pain. Every night I wake up repeatedly because I hurt. Help.

Pain disrupts sleep. Acute pain from surgery, a really bad sore throat, even a twisted ankle or knee can make it hard to fall asleep. Rolling over on a bad shoulder can be a painful reminder to make an appointment with your orthopedic surgeon.

Chronic pain is even worse, chronically disrupting sleep. Insomnia makes the pain worse, which worsens sleep, and so on... Depression is associated with chronic pain. Sleep issues compound depression. You can see where this is leading. So what to do? Control your pain as best you can and your sleep will also improve.

Narcotics, and medications like them, are often necessary for short and long-term pain. Used correctly, they provide relief with relatively few side effects. But abnormal sleep is one of the unwanted effects. Pain pills induce sleep very quickly. But narcotized sleep is not very restorative with less deep and dream (REM) sleep. If you need chronic, daily narcotics for your pain, you can adjust to the abnormal sleep, but it is never perfect. If you are lucky enough to be able to stop taking chronic pain meds, withdrawal insomnia is common. While there is not a perfect answer, sleep is probably better when you are not in pain every night.

Antidepressants are also useful for pain. It is not clear exactly how they work, but they do improve pain, and the Depression and Anxiety that often accompanies pain. Just like narcotics, antidepressants can negatively impact sleep. Brain chemical receptors that control mood and anxiety are also involved in sleep regulation. Antidepressant medications assert their effect through those same chemicals. The sleep effects vary widely. Some make you sleepier. Some wake you up and keep you from sleeping well. You may not have completely normal sleep on antidepressants, but again it is probably better than having untreated pain and Depression.

Neurontin® (gabapentin) is one of the most commonly prescribed drugs for pain. How it works is unclear, but it is a valuable tool in the fight against some of the worst chronic pain syndromes. Like all of the other medication for pain, there is an impact on sleep. But this time the effect is positive. Neurontin® (gabapentin) does not make you feel drowsy during the day and it increases deep sleep stages. Finally, a medication that helps pain and sleep. Neurontin® (gabapentin) is best used to treat nerve pain. If you have shingles or neuropathy from diabetes, this is a good choice.

Being disabled by pain and unable to sleep is not a healthy situation. Pain medications are very powerful and have side effects. One must weigh the risks and benefits of this or any treatment. Finding that balance between pain control, sleep, and daytime function is difficult but possible. Working with a pain specialist is often your best bet.

Q. My wife has Fibromyalgia. She miserable with the pain and can't sleep through the night. What can be done to help her?

Fibromyalgia is the poster child for pain and sleep disturbance. Because of this disease, your wife senses pain, and all unpleasant stimuli, much more intensely than you and me. **(Ceko)** The cause of Fibromyalgia remains a mystery. Unfortunately it is relatively common, present in 2% of the US population. It affects women six times more often than men. **(Arnold)**

There is more to her story than just pain, though. Fibromyalgia is a systemic disease that impacts every aspect of your wife's life. An easy mnemonic to remember the myriad of symptoms caused by Fibromyalgia is "FIBRO." "F" stands for Fibrofog (memory and mental clarity issues) and the Fatigue that comes with it. "I" refers to Insomnia. "B" means the Blues or depression. "R" stands for Rigidity. (This harkens back an old-fashioned name for Fibromyalgia: "Stiff Man Syndrome.") And "O" stands for Ouch. **(Boomershine)** A Fibromyalgia specialist, often a Rheumatologist, should coordinate treatment. **(Hauser)**

So what can be done to help your wife? Lots of things have been suggested from spa treatments to exercise therapy to hypnosis to tai chi to traditional Chinese medicine to psychotherapy to acupuncture to herbs to anti-seizure medications to antidepressants to antipsychotic medications. There is no one-size-fits-all treatment yet. And cure remains elusive. The one FDA approved medication for treatment is Lyrica® (pregabalin). Fortunately, Lyrica® (pregabalin) also helps with sleep by decreasing the time to fall asleep and consolidating and deepening slow wave sleep, which is pretty awesome. **(Boomershine)**

If, despite treatment, she is still having trouble with sleep, the usual sleep aids are helpful. Melatonin may help her fall sleep and might also reduce other symptoms of fibromyalgia. **(Hussein)** Ambien® (zolpidem) or other sleeper medications may help her fall and stay asleep,too. A good night's sleep will help reduce the severity of her symptoms. **(Bennett)**

Lung disease

Breathing has a Circadian Rhythmicity (see Chapter 7, Circadian Rhythm Disorders) to it, varying with the time of the day just like most every other bodily function. If you are having lung problems, sleep does not offer a break. In fact, some lung problems will worsen after sundown and wreak havoc on your sleep.

Q. I have had asthma since I was a kid and seem to be struggling more at night than I used to. Why is that and what should I do about it?

Asthma is a chronic inflammatory disease of the lungs. When the small airways (bronchioles) are irritated they constrict and air doesn't flow well. The result is wheezing, which is the sound of air whistling through those narrow channels. Keeping an asthmatic's bronchioles open and lungs fully inflated during the day is hard enough. It is even tougher at night. Airway irritability and inflammation increase at night due to hormone fluctuations. Heartburn (acid reflux or GERD), which is common at night, can potentially make it even worse. To top it off, breathing is less deep and frequent during sleep. Thus, asthmatics are common late night

151

frequent fliers in the Emergency Room.

If you are struggling to breathe at night you will also struggle to sleep. Awakening frequently causes daytime sleepiness, yes. But, worsening nighttime lung function is linked to a disproportionately high number of asthma deaths that occur during sleep. This is not just a sleep disruption issue. **(Cattaral)**

So the best answer to your question is another question: how well treated is your asthma? If you have had a change for the worse, sit down with your primary care or pulmonary doctor to talk about your asthma therapy. Something has triggered your recent struggle, like an allergy or a sinus or lung infection. Adjusting your medications may be all that is needed.

Q. I have been diagnosed with Obstructive Sleep Apnea and find that my asthma is now much worse. Is there a relationship between the two problems?

Sleep Apnea can worsen your asthma. Conversely, if asthmatic symptoms persist despite good medical treatment, particularly at night, undiagnosed Sleep Apnea may be the cause. The association between OSA and asthma is not entirely clear. It may be that the strain on the lungs during an apnea event triggers wheezing. It could be the hormonal and systemic stressors caused by untreated Sleep Apnea are the causes. Acid reflux, that can initiate bronchospasm, is worse during an apnea. **(Teodorescu)** Your asthma is becoming hard to control. Your Sleep Apnea may be the cause.

Fortunately, treatment of your Sleep Apnea helps quite a bit. Successful OSA treatment decreases acid reflux and reduces the stress and strain on the lungs. Positive airway pressure therapy (CPAP) helps to keep the airways open. It also may make your breathing easier during the day. **(Pellegrino)** More to come on this topic as research progresses.

Q. My mother has idiopathic pulmonary fibrosis (IPF) and is really tired all of the time. Is the lung condition disrupting her sleep?

Yes. IPF is a distressing and destructive disease in which the lungs progressively stiffen until breathing is no longer possible. As the disease progresses breathing takes more and more work. Blood oxygen levels also drop. This is bad enough during the day. At night disrupted and ineffective sleep is common. The result is excessive daytime sleepiness. All of this wreaks havoc on your mother's quality of life. **(Krishnan) (Rasche)**

There is no known uniformly successful therapy for IPF. Providing extra oxygen at night may help with the restfulness of her sleep. Unfortunately the best we can hope for is to stabilize the disease and provide comfort.

Q. I have emphysema from years of smoking. Is that why my sleep is a mess?

Emphysema and Chronic Bronchitis together comprise the diagnosis of Chronic Obstructive Pulmonary Disease (COPD). These two are lumped together because smoking is a common cause. Emphysema describes lung breakdown and stiffness with hyperinflation. Chronic Bronchitis is defined by chronic lung infection that causes inflammation, stiffness, and excessive production of mucus.

You are not alone. Most people (75%) with COPD have disrupted sleep. There are several reasons for sleep disturbance.

The effort required for breathing with diseased lungs makes going to and staying asleep difficult. COPD also causes chronically low blood oxygen levels. Breathing less deeply and less frequently at night makes that even worse. And then there is your persistent, consistent, intrusive, and annoying cough. In the middle of the night it can really disrupt your sleep. And of, course, decreased sleep is accompanied by daytime sleepiness, depressed mood, and poor quality of life.

Treatment of your lung disease, no matter which brand of COPD you have, is about the only tool we have to help your sleep. Inhaled medications can decrease phlegm production and increase airflow by dilating lung passages. Providing extra oxygen overnight may also improve the quality of your sleep. **(Augusti)**

Q. What is this "Overlap Syndrome" my doctor tells me I have?

Overlap Syndrome is a combination of Chronic Obstructive

153

Pulmonary Disease (COPD) with Obstructive Sleep Apnea. Not a good mix. First, your lungs don't function well, inefficiently delivering oxygen and blowing off carbon dioxide. Add in Sleep Apnea, during which you stop breathing at night. Double whammy.

I'll be blunt; you have a higher risk of dying in the night if you have both Sleep Apnea and COPD. Apnea makes the underlying lung disease that much worse.

You need to maximize your lung capacity with an aggressive regimen of medicines, inhalers, and even physical therapy. **(Ezzie)** It is also possible to deliver extra oxygen through the CPAP machine, if needed. Overlap Syndrome is serious. So treating you with CPAP may save your life. Make sure your doctor gets you what you need to protect you from both sides of this disease. (If you need info on Sleep Apnea and CPAP, go to Chapter 5).

Cardiovascular disease

Heart conditions are often worse during sleep. Twenty percent of heart attacks and 15% of sudden cardiac deaths in the United States occur at night. **(Lavery)** Sleep disorders may increase your cardiac risk. So, if you are not careful, danger may be lurking in the night.

Q. My cardiologist seems to think that I am at risk for another heart attack in my sleep. She said I am probably a "non-dipper." What the heck is she talking about?

Most people drop their blood pressure by 10-20% when asleep at night. They are "dippers" whose blood pressure is doing what it is supposed to do. **(Routledge)** Dropping blood pressure and a slowed heart rate during sleep are likely a protective mechanisms, allowing the heart to rest and restore like the rest of the body. **(Penzel)**

Your blood pressure may not go down at night, thus the "non-dipper" designation. This can be a real problem. You are at increased risk for heart attack because your heart doesn't get a break overnight. It has to work just as hard while you are asleep as when you are awake. **(Penzel)** To take the risk out of falling asleep, and to avoid the risk of a nighttime cardiac event, make sure your blood pressure is controlled 24/7

Q. I had a 24 hour heart monitor because of palpitations and they saw a lot of more issues with my heart while I was asleep. Why is that?

Sleep can be very stressful on an already sick heart. A couple of normal nighttime conditions may be putting your already palpitating heart at risk for more problems.

First, the heart normally slows during sleep at night. The slower nighttime rate allows what we call "escape" beats. A faster daytime heartbeat usually keeps those extra abnormal beats from sneaking through and triggering all kinds of mayhem.

Second, to make matters worse, heart rate and blood pressure go up in REM sleep. This sleep stage is a very unstable time. Significant cardiac variability is normal. In the extreme case adrenalin speeds the heart in a fight or flight reaction. These are treacherous waters for a person who has a sick heart already. **(Verrier)**

What to do? Well you can't stay awake all of the time. But, you can make sure to take your blood pressure and heart rhythm medicine. If you have any suspicion that you may have Obstructive Sleep Apnea get yourself checked out. (See Chapter 5 if you need more information on OSA.) You have enough heart problems without that added strain. If you do have OSA, CPAP (continuous positive airway pressure) may save your life.

Q. My grandfather has Congestive Heart Failure and he is struggling every night. Why is that and what can we do to help?

"Heart failure" literally means that the heart is failing to pump blood to the body and the lungs efficiently. The consequences of a failing heart are widespread and disruptive in the daytime and at night. During the day, since his heart is so weak, fluid accumulates in the legs due to gravity. At night, when he lies down and elevates his legs, that fluid is released into the circulation to wreak havoc and disrupt his sleep. Let me diagram the chain of events for you...

155

DAYTIME
Poor blood circulation due to heart failing to
pump well
↓
Fluid collects in the ankles and feet because of
gravity
↓
NIGHTTIME
Feet are up when he lies down and ankle/feet
fluid re-enters the blood stream
↓
Increased fluid in the blood stream makes the
heart work harder
↓
Fluid now accumulates in the lungs →   Increasing blood flow and fluid
↓   delivered to the kidneys
Lungs become stiff = hard to breathe   ↓

More urine = frequent
nighttime urination

↘   ↙

POOR SLEEP!

It gets even worse from here. In late stage heart failure a
nighttime breathing pattern develops that further messes with sleep.
It is called Cheyne-Stokes breathing, or less charitably the "death
rattle." This pattern is characterized by increasing speed and depth
of breathing (hyperpnea) followed by slowing and then cessation of
breathing (apnea). Breathing then starts up again repeating the same
pattern. Cheyne-Stokes is depicted on the graph below:

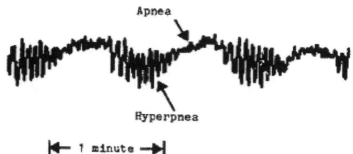

Those fast deep breathing periods are the equivalent of
panting and often disrupt sleep.

156

Finally, heart failure can cause intermittent awakenings with a sense of suffocating shortness of breath. This is called Paroxysmal (meaning it occurs randomly) Nocturnal (nighttime) Dyspnea (difficulty breathing), or PND for short. **(Mukerji)** The exact mechanism of PND is not entirely clear. It is most likely related to heart dysfunction and fluid accumulation in the lungs.

So your grandfather's heart failure is very disruptive to his sleep on many levels. The best answer for helping him rest better is to make sure he is following his doctor's recommendations and taking all prescribed treatments. If he is still struggling, a return visit to the cardiologist is needed to figure out why he isn't responding better. If his heart failure is better controlled his sleep should improve.

Kidney and Urinary Tract disease

Like most medical problems, kidney and urinary problems can influence sleep. Some of these problems are simple and logical. Some of them are a little more obscure.

Q. I have to pee all of the time, but especially in the middle of the night. Why is that?

If you are a man, you need to first get your prostate checked. Not real exciting, I know. But if you have a "going" problem, as the commercial says, you may go so frequently at night that you can't get a good night's sleep. Your prostate gland sits along he path of your urethra (the tube leading from the bladder to the outside world.) If the prostate enlarges it narrows the urethra and limits flow. Limited flow causes pressure to build in the bladder. Increased pressure in the bladder instigates the urge to pee. In the extreme case over time, flow blockage causes your bladder to blow up like a balloon and incompletely empty. When this occurs the muscles are stretched out and no longer capable of squeezing the urine past the prostate, which becomes a medical emergency. **(Anacoli-Israel)** If this sounds familiar, you probably need to visit a Urologist to define the severity of the problem and determine a medical or surgical treatment approach.

Women have bladder problems that unsettle sleep, too. If you suffer from Chronic Interstitial Cystitis/Painful Bladder Syndrome (chronic irritation of the bladder) sleep can suffer. Over 1 million American women (and a few men too) are affected. Pelvic pain, urgency to pee, multiple small volume releases, and lower abdominal pressure are common symptoms. The chronic annoying bladder irritation interrupts falling asleep, causes middle of the night awakenings, and leads to earlier rising. **(Chelimsky)** Multiple treatments are available, including bladder exercises, dietary modifications, the introduction of medications directly into the bladder, and oral medications. Elmiron® (pentosan) is commonly prescribed to improve the health of the bladder lining. **(French)**

Q. My husband has been a diabetic for years and now is in kidney failure. He is on dialysis and doing better, but just can't seem to get any good sleep. He is exhausted all of the time. What can we do to help him?

Kidney failure wreaks havoc on sleep. And renal dialysis patients are the poster children for this problem, with 61% reporting difficulty sleeping. **(Al-Jahdali)** Not only does he feel bad because his kidneys aren't working well, he is also sleep deprived. Unfortunately there isn't much to do about it. Even successful dialysis doesn't seem to help. The sleep issue is a complicated one. Kidney failure causes systemic issues that are difficult to improve. Making sure that your husband has adequate time for sleep and minimal distractions at night, just like anyone, is about the best one can do.

Q. Since my kidneys went out I can't seem to settle down at night and go to sleep. The weirdest thing is that it feels like I have snakes running up and down under the skin of my legs. When I get out of bed and walk it feels better. But as soon as I lie down again it comes back. This is driving me nuts. Am I?

You are definitely not nuts. You are describing classic Restless Legs Syndrome (RLS), which is very common in people with kidney failure. (For a more complete discussion of RLS, go to Chapter 9, Movements That Wake You Up.) It is also very disruptive to falling sleep. RLS occurs in 20% or more of people on dialysis. **(Parish)** It is linked to iron deficiency in otherwise healthy people.

It is a mystery why kidney failure and RLS often occur together. Some experts think that both iron deficiency and kidney failure result in the same brain dysfunction that ultimately leads to the symptoms. Iron supplementation is the first line of therapy. If that is not curative, medications that increase brain dopamine levels (Requip® (ropinirole) and Mirapex® pramipexole)) often help. **(Brindini)**

Gastrointestinal Problems

Q. I wake up with burning in my throat, coughing and choking, every night. It is really scary, not to mention that I can't sleep. How can I make this stop?

Gastroesophageal reflux disease (or GERD as it is affectionately know) is common at night. Most everyone has experienced the discomfort of heartburn at one time or another. Belching, burning, chest pain and pressure, and stomach pain, are bad enough when you are awake. In the middle of the night it is even worse.

Most of the time you have done it to yourself. Eating the Fiesta Grande Mexican Plate #8 right before bedtime really revs up acid production. When you lie down, gravity can't keep the jalapenos in your stomach where they belong. The second time around is not nearly as enjoyable.

Sometimes acid reflux is a chronic problem. It doesn't matter what or when you eat, you regurgitate.

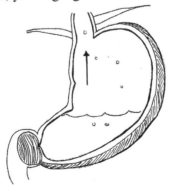

Julia Argent

159

Avoiding instigators of acid reflux is your first step. Alcohol, Nicotine, and Caffeine all relax the muscle sphincter at the bottom of the esophagus that should keep stomach stuff in the stomach. So having a cup of coffee after dinner, a nightcap, or one last cigarette, may trigger GERD. Prevention is worth an ounce of cure. Be careful what and when you eat/drink/smoke. Identifying and avoiding your GERD trigger(s) is the easiest and most effective treatment.

If diet and lifestyle changes haven't fixed your heartburn, you probably need medication. I don't recommend the routine use of remedies like TUMS and Milk of Magnesia. They act directly to neutralize stomach acid, but the effect is transient. There are much more effective over-the-counter medications that work better if you need more than just occasional temporary relief.

Famotidine, Ranitidine, and Cimetidine (Axid®, Zantac®, and Tagamet®, respectively) work to block nerve impulse to the stomach that incite acid production during meals. Hindering that message results in less stomach acid. These are safe for long-term use and have few side effects.

The most effective drugs are the "proton pump inhibitors." They directly stop the stomach cells that produce acid. Over-the-counter Prilosec®, Zegerid® (omeprazole) and Prevacid® (lansoprazole), at half the prescription strength, are usually sufficient for most people. Prescription strength medications include Dexilent® (dexlansoprazole), Nexium® (esomeprazole), Protonix® (pantoprazole) and Aciphex® (rabeprozole) to name a few. OTC meds carry a recommendation that you limit use to 2 weeks or consult a physician, which is reasonable. But long-term use rarely has digestive side effects. As an aside, women need to be careful with chronic use due to the potential to worsen osteoporosis. For the most part these are great medications.

If these drugs don't work, further evaluation is in order. It may be that you have a more serious stomach infection, ulcer, or even a tumor. You may need a procedure (upper GI endoscopy) to take a look at your esophagus and stomach. A visit to a Gastroenterologist is your next step.

Neurological Disease

Any disease that affects the brain can affect sleep. There are a multitude of real and significant neurological disorders. While all of those diseases are important, the focus here is on the most common ones.

Q. My mother has Alzheimer's and her sleep is all over the place. She is up all night and naps frequently during the day. Is this to be expected with Alzheimer's disease?

It is heartbreaking for you to watch your mother's mental capacity diminish, and with it her ability to take care of herself. You are not alone. Alzheimer's and other forms of dementia are becoming more prevalent in the US. It is estimated that over 5 million people in the US have Alzheimer's now and that number will increase as the population ages. Dementia related sleep disruption has many causes: brain dysfunction, medication effects, and poor sleep hygiene due to mental degeneration. Sleep Apnea is also a frequent co-occurrence.

Treating an Alzheimer's patient with sleep problems is complicated. Any medication that causes sleepiness can potentially worsen her dementia and confusion. Sedatives, antidepressants, and even her Alzheimer's meds can cause drowsiness. But, treating her insomnia and depression/anxiety can also improve her Alzheimer's symptoms by providing for a better night of sleep. It is a difficult balance to strike.

Rozerem® (ramelteon) is a Melatonin mimic with low side effects that shows promise to help Insomnia associated with Alzheimer's. It lacks the sedating side effects of other medications while improving sleep. For some reason, Melatonin itself is not so effective. **(Deschenes)**

Because pharmacologic treatment of dementia-related sleep problems is so difficult, non-medical approaches are really important. Strict Sleep Hygiene is the key. During the daytime, mental stimulation that encourages engagement and alertness, and exposure to daytime light (ideally sunlight), both stimulate wakefulness. Daytime physical activity increases energy, strength, endurance, and decreases fall risk. These activities help align sleep

161

and wake timing (Circadian Rhythms) with night and day. Napping opportunities need to be limited to early in the day so that she is tired and ready for bed in the evening.

The nighttime sleep environment must be safe, dark, and quiet. Aligning schedules with family and friends improves sleep. **(Martin)**

Adjusting your Grandmother's sleep wake schedules may make a real difference, enough so that medications aren't necessary.

Q. I have been diagnosed with Lou Gehrig's disease and my sleep has gone down hill with the rest of my body. What can I do to get a good night's sleep?

ALS (Amyotrophic Lateral Sclerosis in medicalese, Lou Gehrig's disease in normal language) is a rare, devastating disease that progressively weakens muscles. Sleep is a casualty of ALS because of declining breathing muscle strength.

During normal breathing, the chest wall expands outward and the diaphragm contracts downward to pull air into the lungs. In REM sleep (or dream sleep) all muscles, except the diaphragm, are purposefully inhibited from moving. Because of ALS, your diaphragm doesn't move. So, during REM sleep you can't breathe - because none of those breathing muscles are working. REM sleep is essentially eliminated from your night because you have to wake up to breathe repeatedly during that sleep stage. Sleep without REM is not restful, restorative sleep. That is why you are tired. **(Arnulf)**

So what can be done to help? In the extreme case a home ventilator, called Non-Invasive Positive Pressure Ventilation (NIPPV), can keep you breathing at night. NIPPV comes with a set up similar to a CPAP for Obstructive Sleep Apnea: a mask covering your nose +/- mouth connected to an air pump. The machine senses airflow. If you stop breathing during REM it bumps up the pressure to push a breath into your lungs. As you become progressively weaker, you may need the ventilator function no matter what stage of sleep you are in. Stephen Hawkings, the famous British physicist, has ALS and needs a ventilator awake or asleep. He has been alive and productive for years this way. Not surprisingly you are more awake and function better mentally when treated with NIPPV. **(Newsom-Davis)**

Unfortunately we can't yet change the course of ALS. Hopefully researchers will someday find a cure.

Q. I have these horrible headaches that only hit me while I am asleep. What can be done?

Hypnic Headaches, also known as Alarm Clock Headaches, are disturbing and disruptive but also easily treated. **(Ganguly)** These rare headaches wake you up in the early morning hours, probably during REM sleep. Unlike migraines, you feel no nausea or sensitivity to light. The pain lasts from a half to several hours and then goes away.

Treatment is initiated if you have these headaches frequently. Lithobid® (lithium), the same stuff used to treat bipolar disease, is your best option. Indocin® (indomethacin) has also been used for treatment with variable success. **(De Simone)**

Q. My Parkinson's Disease is getting progressively worse and my sleep is going with it. Why is that and how can I get a good night's sleep?

This is unfortunately very common. Non-restorative sleep has a negative impact on your Parkinson's and every other part of your life. Most people with Parkinson's have sleep problems for many reasons:

1. Parkinson's Disease is caused by a decrease in dopamine, one of the brain's chemical messengers that control movement. Because Parkinson's makes you stiff it is difficult to turn over in bed, which can lead to pain from lying in the same position all night. Tremors and other involuntary movements make it difficult to relax and fall asleep. Dementia and Depression, both of which are associated with sleep problems, are common too.

2. Medications to treat Parkinson's disease increase brain dopamine, which helps to relieve stiffness and tremor. However, those drugs also are associated with vivid dreaming and even nightmares. **(Menza)**

3. Having REM Behavior Disorder (RBD) (as discussed in Chapter 11, REM Associate Parasomnias) doesn't always predict the development of Parkinson's. Having Parkinson's does not require

RBD. But they often go hand in hand. One of the hallmark characteristics in REM sleep is the almost complete inhibition of muscle movement. If you have RBD, your muscles are active no matter what stage of sleep you are in. So it is possible for you to act out your dreams, which is disturbing to sleep and potentially dangerous. **(Trotti)** Treatment is usually easy; a mild sedative (Klonopin® (clonazepam)) typically alleviates the symptoms with minimal side effects.

4. Restless Legs Syndrome (RLS - as discussed in Chapter 9, Movements That Wake You Up) is also common in Parkinson's disease, much more so than the general population. Having creepy crawlies in your legs makes it hard to fall asleep. There is an association between iron deficiency and RLS. Blood tests to determine iron and ferritin levels are needed. If you are deficient, treatment with iron supplementation works well. If that isn't your issue, you are not out of luck. Fortunately, both Parkinson's and RLS are treated with medications that increase dopamine in the brain. **(Ondo)**

Considering your diagnosis, having disrupted sleep is no surprise. Make sure that your Parkinson's therapy is fine tuned to decrease rigidity and tremors. Also, make sure you don't have a more common diagnosis, like Sleep Apnea, that needs treatment. And just like everyone else, make sure you are prepared for bed (e.g. good Sleep Hygiene as described in Chapter 2, Advice for Smarter Sleep) so you can get to sleep easily. Be active during the day and limit naps. If you are still struggling, sleep medications like Ambien® (zolpidem) may be necessary.

Epilepsy

Q. Our son has had seizures for a couple of years after a closed head injury. Except for continued seizures, he has recovered in every other way. He has been on a variety of medications but is still seizing and tired during the day. What can be done?

Seizures result from the activation of abnormal brain pathways that lead to uncontrolled movements and/or sensory experiences. Insomnia and sleep problems accompany epilepsy much more than in the general population for a variety of reasons. Your son's daytime sleepiness might just result from altered brain function due to his injury. His brain may not yet control and regulate sleep well. But he may be having nighttime seizures that interrupt sleep that he doesn't even know about. These occur in about 25% of people with epilepsy.

Further complicating matters is the sleepiness side effect of the very anti-epileptic medications used to control seizures. (More on this in the Medications and Sleep Chapter 17.) Your son's sleep may be poor if is experiencing the anxiety and depression that often go along with Epilepsy. Mood disorders often lead to Insomnia regardless of cause. **(Beyenburg)** So there are a LOT of reasons he may be sleepy during the day. **(deHaas)**

Don't overlook more mundane sleep problems either. Just because you have Epilepsy doesn't mean that you can't have other unrelated difficulties like Sleep Apnea or Restless Legs Syndrome.

Finally, sleep deprivation increases the likelihood of seizures. More seizures lead to more sleep disruption. It is a vicious cycle. If necessary he may need to undergo an overnight sleep study with extended brain wave (EEG) monitoring to determine if he truly is having nighttime seizures.

What to do? The good news is that seizure control improves sleep. He will also eventually adjust to any sedating side effects of antiseizure medication. Make sure that your son and his neurologist are working together to maximize his therapy. **(Malow)**

Q. My husband has had a stroke and, in addition to all of the other problems he is facing, can't seem to get a good night's sleep. Is this common?

A stroke (or Cerebrovascular Accident - CVA) is a brain injury due either to a bleed into, or a clot that blocks blood flow to a part of, the brain. Either way blood flow is interrupted causing damage. Stroke victims have varying degrees of impairment, depending on what area of the brain is injured (movement, vision, hearing, etc.)

One thing almost all stroke victims have trouble with is Insomnia. Sleep stages and consolidation of sleep are affected early on after a CVA. With time, as the brain recovers, so does sleep

165

control and coordination. And recovery of normal sleep is associated with better functional recovery. **(Vock) (Schuiling)** Daytime sleepiness worsens the effect of stroke and interferes with rehabilitation efforts. Also, Depression is common after a stroke, which is a major cause of Insomnia (see Insomnia, Chapter 3 for more information). **(Teroni)**

If your husband can avoid medication for sleep he will probably fare better. Good Sleep Hygiene (Advice for Smarter Sleep in Chapter 2 can fill you in on this topic) is really important. Make sure he has a dark, comfortable, quiet, safe, and familiar sleep environment. Keep his bedtime very consistent. Discourage naps to insure he is ready to sleep at night. Exercise and daytime activity are helpful to get him tired for sleep at night. Also, daylight exposure encourages alignment of his internal clock/Circadian Rhythms to day night schedules.

If non-medical approaches are ineffective, medications are an option until he heals and recovers better brain function. Prescribing a sedative must be done with care and deliberation. A tranquilizer hangover can make him even sleepier than his current situation.

Q. My wife has Multiple Sclerosis and sleeps for hours. Is this normal with MS?

She is like most people with MS; tiredness is very common. Why MS predisposes to poor sleep and daytime sleepiness isn't clear. It may have to do with the immune problems that cause MS in the first place. Depression and other sleep diagnoses, including Sleep Apnea, also disturb sleep frequently.

First make sure she doesn't have any unrelated medical problems, like anemia, Depression, or thyroid problems. Also, she may need a sleep medicine consultation to look for other sleep problems. If all else is ok, we can treat her with the wake promoters Provigil® (modafinil) or Nuvigil® (armodafinil) to brighten up her daytime. **(Braley)**

Cancer

Q. My grandmother is dying from cancer. Her sleep is really a problem. What can we do to help her rest?

People afflicted by cancer have much more Insomnia and daytime sleepiness than healthy people for many reasons. Depression and mood disorders, that are strongly associated with Insomnia, often accompany a diagnosis of malignancy. Cancer therapies themselves disrupt sleep by causing pain, nausea, weakness, and fatigue. Having a malignant tumor normally saps energy, disrupts bodily functions, and impacts comfort, depending on the location and what it directly affects. **(Parish)** Overall, cancer causes daytime fatigue regardless of sleep issues. **(Campos)**

Your grandmother's sleep issues need a comprehensive approach. Fatigue and sleepiness impact her ability to recover. She needs to have an open mind and approach this with all options available. There is great utility in medications to relieve pain and sedate her for sleep. Non-medical therapies have real impact too. Psychological counseling to help her cope with the disease is key. Music, imagery, meditation, and even hypnosis are useful interventions to help her mind and body improve daytime and nighttime function. **(Kwekkeboom)** Cancer centers and oncologists (cancer doctors) are well aware of their patients' sleep problems and will provide ready access to helpful resources.

Infection

Q. It seems that every time I get a cold or stomach bug I end up in bed asleep for hours, and it doesn't mess up my sleep like a nap would when I am well. So why am I so sleepy when I am sick?

Being sick is stressful, which wears you out. But there is more to the sleepiness than that. Your immune system reacts to infections in a very complicated and sophisticated way. Two of the thousands of chemicals that immune cells produce to fight off infections, IL-1β (interleukin-1 beta) and TNF-α (tumor necrosis factor-alpha), cause sleepiness. This is a normal part of our reaction to being infected. Sleep is also one of the most important components of healing from an illness.

Q. My daughter has had HIV for several years. After getting over the shock and depression, she had gotten on with her life. However she doesn't sleep very well now. Is this part of HIV or should we treat this just like anyone else with a sleep issue?

Sleep problems plague most people who are infected with HIV, women more than men. Insomnia is common, causing fatigue and lack of energy. **(Lee2)** High viral counts (with low white cell counts) indicating active infection may cause her to feel sleepy too. Ironically, treatment with anti-retroviral medications is also associated with sleep problems. **(Lee1)**

Getting a good night's sleep is essential to your daughter's health. Depression and Anxiety are common accompaniments to HIV/AIDS. So make sure she has access to good mental health resources. **(Junqueira)** Good Sleep Hygiene (see Advice for Smarter Sleep, Chapter 2) makes a difference. If necessary, melatonin or even prescription sedative medications are useful.

Q. I have a severe case of Lyme Disease and my doctor says some of my sleeping problems can be blamed on the infection. Is this true and can I get better?

Lyme Disease is an unusual infection contracted by a bite from a deer tick. It is a complex disease with a wide range of affects and severity that vary from person to person. Initial manifestations of Lyme Disease range from a rash to meningitis to heart problems to arthritis. If you have central nervous system/brain infection, your sleep may be affected. **(Kalish)** A multitude of sleep problems are reported to be associated with Lyme Disease, including Restless Legs Syndrome and Insomnia. **(Parish)** Fortunately, with successful treatment of Lyme Disease, even if severe, comes improved neurological problems, including sleep. **(Logigian)**

Chapter 15: Psychiatric Problems and Sleep

Psychiatric diseases are finally being recognized as medical problems of brain function, not character flaws and moral weaknesses. Better understanding of brain chemical abnormalities that account for psychiatric illness has lead to more effective treatments.

It is clear that sleep and psychiatric problems are tightly linked. The same neurotransmitter misregulation that causes psychiatric illness also negatively affects sleep. Understanding brain chemistry, and the chemistry of mental disorders, will provide a better understanding of associated sleep problems. **(Harvey)**

Depression

Q. Depression runs in my family and I find myself having trouble sleeping. I know that my depressed relatives suffered from sleep issues, too. Should I see my doctor about depression because my sleep is slowly and surely deteriorating?

You are correct that people diagnosed with real, medical Depression (not just sadness) have a lot of sleep problems. Most have some form of Insomnia. On the one hand, they may have trouble going to sleep, staying asleep, or awake up too early. On the other hand, some depressed people have Hypersomnia (they are sleepy all of the time) as part of their mood disorder. Many depressed people had problems with sleep long before their Depression diagnosis. To muddle the picture a bit, people with sleep disorders (like Sleep Apnea – Chapter 4, Restless Legs Syndrome and/or Periodic Limb Movement Disorder – Chapter 9, and Narcolepsy – Chapter 13) often also have Depression. So which came first, the chicken (sleep issues) or the egg (Depression)? One thing is certain; it is difficult to overcome Major Depression if sleep disturbances are not also addressed. **(Franzen)**

Advanced Sleep Phase Syndrome (ASPS), a Circadian Rhythm Disorder (which I encourage you to read about in Chapter 7), may be closely tied to the sleep issues in Depression. To review, people who have ASPS feel the need to sleep earlier than most. They have the same sleep mechanisms that a "normal" person does (melatonin release, sleep stage achievement, sleep time, and awake time); they just do this at an earlier hour. Research demonstrates that depressed people with Insomnia have similar sleep physiology as people with Advanced Sleep Phase Syndrome (including patterns of body temperature fluctuations, dream sleep timing, and timed hormonal releases). So is there a connection? Maybe so. A genetic link may yet be uncovered. **(Lamont)**

What does this mean for you? It is hard to say. People with Depression often report Insomnia that predates the onset of their mood problems. **(Franzen)** It is also true that Major Depression runs in families genetically. **(Lohoff)**

You are definitively at risk for Depression just because you are not sleeping well and you have a family history. Be vigilant about your sleep and your moods. If you are starting to be depressed, your sleep is deteriorating further, and your relationships are suffering, seek help. Treatment of Insomnia improves Depression. **(Lamont)** Treatment of Depression with medications and individual psychotherapy helps with sleep issues. **(Kupfer)** Early intervention is key to keep you from falling into the abyss of Major Depression.

Q. My wife has Postpartum Depression. The worse her sleep becomes, the more her mood deteriorates. She is breastfeeding so I can't help feed the baby at night. This feels like a downward spiral that I can't stop. What can I do to help?

New moms have it rough. Newborns are screaming, needy, unregulated, bundles of joy. They demand care 24/7, and most of that care falls on Mom, especially if she is breastfeeding. So her sleep is naturally going to be disrupted. Other sleep disturbances also occur due to the hormonal rebalancing that inevitably occurs in the transition back from pregnancy. Sleep deficiency plus hormonal turmoil sets up many women for psychiatric problems.

Postpartum Depression (PPD) occurs in up to 12% of new mothers. Life is a living hell with a new baby and despair. This is real, full-blown Depression: decreased interest in life (and her baby), persistent sadness, weight loss, anxiety, loss of energy and ability to concentrate, and even suicidal thoughts. **(Posmontier)** The impact on the woman is bad enough, but the baby suffers too. And, as you

170

have described, this affects the whole family. When PPD hits, things can deteriorate very quickly.

Even without a baby, women who have bad sleep are more prone to be depressed. And, women with Depression are prone to have disrupted and ineffectual sleep. **(Dørheim)** Other risk factors for developing PPD include Depression before pregnancy, other personal or family psychiatric problems, poverty, and lack of support at home. **(Posmontier)** There is more to Post Partum Depression than just being sleep deprived.

Moms with PPD need help, lots of it. Her Obstetrician and the baby's Pediatrician should be able to provide referrals to mental health professionals. As with all forms of Depression, counseling is a mainstay of treatment. There are natural concerns about the use of antidepressant medications (particularly the SSRIs – see Chapter 17, Medications and Sleep for a discussion of how these drugs affect sleep in general) during pregnancy and breastfeeding. The good news is that most of those medications are relatively safe for the baby. The impact of untreated Depression on the health of the mother and the baby generally outweighs the minimal risk. **(Meltzer-Brody)**

As a concerned Dad, you need to help as much as you can. Take night duty as often as you can to allow your wife to get some much needed sleep. Having pumped breast milk available for middle of a night bottle-feeds takes some of the pressure off of her. It is sometimes necessary to stop breastfeeding completely, despite the obvious health advantages to the baby and mother, so she can sleep and recover. Your child will be ok either way. A loving, stable, and emotionally healthy home is the most important thing you and your wife can provide for your child. Do whatever it takes to make that happen for all of you.

Anxiety and Panic Disorders

Q. I have been diagnosed with Generalized Anxiety Disorder and I am a wreck day and night. Help.

Living with Anxiety is miserable. Excessive worry and concern negatively impact concentration, productivity, and every other facet of life. It is surprisingly common. One in four people

171

have significant Anxiety at some point in their lives. **(Staner)**
Making matters worse is the impact on sleep. Racing thoughts and
apprehension make going to, and staying, asleep very difficult.
(Abad)

Anxiety is often cause the cause of Chronic Insomnia. An
inability to sleep leads to tiredness and fatigue. Feeling so tired
increases your worry and anxiety about getting through the day.
Those feelings in turn disrupt sleep at night. It is a vicious cycle.

Treatment is usually a combination of medication and
therapy. Counseling is vital to create understanding and to strategize
approaches for symptom control. Medications, particularly the
modern antidepressants, are useful for the worry and ruminations
that are so disruptive.

Controlling anxiety improves sleep. But on occasion a
prescription sleeping pill is needed, particularly early on until
counseling and antidepressants kick in. **(Staner)** Long-term control
of Anxiety is the goal, returning you to a life uncluttered by
excessive angst and fear. With that comes more normal and restful
sleep. Having to take chronic sedative and anti-anxiety medications
is by no means a failure. It is better to be happy, healthy, and
medicated than suffer chronic anxiety.

**Q. I was in Iraq for 3 tours of duty. I have been diagnosed with
Post Traumatic Stress Disorder (PTSD) at the VA and am
supposed to start treatment. I am a mess and my sleep is even
worse. I just can't relax to go to sleep. Isn't there some pill I can
take?**

Many of our finest young people have served our country in
time of war and struggle when they get home. The stress and strain
of living with death and making it back alive takes a toll. PTSD is
common among returning veterans. It also happens to people after
other traumatic events, like auto accidents, assaults, abuse, and
injuries. The previously experienced trauma is continually relived
while awake and while asleep in the form of nightmares.
(vanLiempt) The vicious circle of nightmares disrupting sleep, that
leads to tiredness and fatigue, which contributes to sleep problems,
that increases the likelihood of nightmares and Insomnia has to be
broken before healing can start.

172

Psychotherapy is a mainstay of treatment for PTSD. However, a medication called Minipress® (prazosin) has found promise in treating Nightmare Disorder, especially when it is due to PTSD. Minipress® (prazosin) works by blocking adrenalin receptors in the brain. Blocking those receptors inhibits the brain's response to PTSD stress leading to better sleep and less nightmares. By improving sleep, some of the strain of the PTSD reaction can be blunted. Combining medication with appropriate therapy is often the best approach.

Q. My son was diagnosed with Panic Disorder (PD) years ago but now is having problems at night. Is this just a nighttime version of his daytime attacks or do we have to worry about another problem?

He has probably developed Nighttime Panic Disorder (NPD). Panic disorder is very common, affecting millions of Americans. These unfortunate souls are occasionally, and sometimes seemingly randomly, gripped with great fear and anxiety about sudden death. Accompanying the terror is a racing heart, dry mouth, chest pain, room spins, and even nausea. Around half of people with PD will have nighttime episodes. Imagine awakening from sleep feeling terrified that death is upon you. (**Abad**)

Even worse is the combination of NPD and Sleep Paralysis. Imagine waking up afraid you may die <u>and</u> not being able to move. It would be awfully hard to go back to sleep after that experience! Unfortunately, this is a fairly common combination. (**Sharpless**) (see Chapter 11, REM Associated Parasomnias, for a closer look at Sleep Paralysis.)

Treatment for Panic Disorder and its nighttime manifestations include counseling and medications, like any anxiety disorder. Having a psychologist or psychiatrist work with your son to help him understand and deal with the frightening symptoms of panic can be very effective. Medications used in conjuction with therapy, like SSRI antidepressants (Luvox® (fluvoxamine), Prozac® (fluoxetine), Paxil® (paroxetine), Celexa® (citalopram), Zoloft® ()) are useful as well. (**Austin**)

Obsessive Compulsive Disorder

Q. My wife has always been a little neurotic, but now has been diagnosed with Obsessive Compulsive Disorder (OCD) and feels like she can't sleep. How can I help her?

OCD is miserable. It can take over your life. Excessive focus on small details or repetitive actions is an attempt to soothe the anxiety that generates the obsession. Those compulsive behaviors drive activities that, if not performed, generate anxiety again. While there are no sleep disturbances that are specific to Obsessive Compulsive Disorder, chronic Insomnia is common. Lack of sleep never makes anything better.

Oddly, there are some people with OCD who feel like Insomniacs when in fact they are sleeping just fine. Sleep State Misperception (as discussed on page in Chapter 3, Sleeplessness – not to be missed reading!) is a misinterpretation of how much sleep a person is actually getting. They are sleeping 7 or 8 hours a night, but say they aren't getting a wink.

Great success has been achieved treating the obsessions and compulsions with antidepressants like Effexor® (venlafaxine). However, counseling and psychotherapy are also useful. Interaction with a mental health professional helps the person with OCD see the bigger picture. Improvement in sleep often follows. **(Abe)** To help your wife sleep, get her OCD treated.

Attention Deficit Hyperactivity Disorder

Q. My husband has been diagnosed with ADHD. He doesn't sleep well and I am worried that if he starts those stimulant medications he really won't sleep. What's the right answer?

Attention Deficit Disorder (ADD) and Attention Deficit Hyperactivity Disorder (ADHD) are increasingly common diagnoses in adults. Up to 12% of kids and 4% of adults are affected. Though they may not have been diagnosed as kids, most of the grown ups probably had problems then as well. **(Meijer)** Difficulty focusing, lack of concentration, and impulsivity, among other things, are very disruptive to relationships and occupational productivity.

People with ADD/ADHD do not have normal sleep. Studies

show that they take longer to fall asleep, have more middle of the night awakenings, and experience less REM sleep. (Sobanski) Worsening ADD/ADHD symptoms cause worsening sleep. And as expected, adding any component of Depression or a mood disorder compounds the problem. (Agarwal)

Treatment of ADHD/ADD usually includes, paradoxically, the use of stimulants. Ritalin®/Concerta® (methylphenidate), Adderall® (amphetamine-dextroamphetamine), and Dexedrine® (dextroamphetamine) are mainstay medications. (Refer to Chapter 17, Medications and Sleep section for more information on how these drugs affect sleep.) If a person without ADD takes one of these they feel hyped up, energetic, anxious, and hyperactive; sort of like what a person with ADD feels like. However, when taken for ADD he feels calmer, more focused, and relaxed. And, if you can get your ADD/ADHD treated you will sleep better. You can fall asleep faster and stay asleep better as compared to sleep off medications. (Sobanski)

Timing is everything, though. If taken too late in the day these stimulant medications can keep him from falling sleep. Dose and timing need to balance the effect on daytime focus with the need for adequate nighttime sleep.

As with any medication, stimulants have other potential side effects. They may cause headaches, loss of appetite, and insomnia even when used appropriately. (Agarwal)

Also, just because you have ADD/ADHD doesn't mean you can't have other sleep problems, like Sleep Apnea, sleep-related movement disorders, or Insomnia. Treating any sleep disorder that might also be disrupting sleep will help with ADD/ADHD symptoms too.

Psychosis

Q. My schizophrenic son is up at all hours. I worry because his lack of sleep seems to make control of his hallucinations much more difficult. What can be done to help him sleep?

A person with active Schizophrenia is said to be Psychotic, meaning they have lost contact with reality. They have delusions (misunderstandings and misguided beliefs about what is happening around them), and hallucinations (sensing sounds, sights, feelings, and even tastes and smells that aren't actually happening). It is a horrific way to live.

Almost all people with psychosis have difficulty falling and staying asleep. Schizophrenics also don't have as much deep sleep, including REM sleep, as compared to someone without Psychosis. **(Kane)** So even if your son gets an uninterrupted night of sleep, he still may not have restorative rest. Schizophrenics also are more often "late night people" which could indicate some sort of sleep timing (Circadian) problems. **(Lamont)** This could explain "Night Owl" behavior often seen in people with psychosis.

Daytime sleepiness due to poor sleep quality and quantity has a big impact on the quality of life experienced by someone with Schizophrenia. Coping skills and happiness are really affected if the disease and its treatment, with anti-psychotic medications, are compounded by sleep problems as well. **(Hofstetter)**

So what to do with the sleep issues is a great question. I am not sure we are at a place where categorical answers can be provided. Every person with psychosis is different and requires a unique and individual approach. Throwing a sedative at the sleep problems associated with Schizophrenia is not the best first step. Good Sleep Hygiene (Chapter 2, Advice for Smarter Sleep) with consistent bedtimes and rise times, a safe and quiet sleep environment, and nap avoidance are really helpful. Low dose Melatonin, daytime bright light exposure, and regular physical activity may all play a part in maintaining good nighttime sleep health. If there is a need for both antipsychotic and sedative medication the psychiatrist and sleep specialist need to work closely to prevent unintended side effects of mixed medications.

As for anyone, good sleep is important for good mental function. Your son's sleep needs to be a priority to help him manage his underlying mental illness.

Q. Bipolar Disease runs in my family and I remember my uncle being up all night even when he was okay mentally. Why do people with this affliction have so much trouble sleeping?

Bipolar Disease, like Schizophrenia, can wreak havoc on a person's life and that of his or her family. Extreme mood swings are disruptive in the extreme. Intense energy, activity, appetite, sexuality, and irresponsibility (Mania) and powerful melancholy, sadness, fatigue, and lack of motivation (Depression) represent the opposite ends of Bipolar Disorder. But, it is not just the extremes that cause problems. People with bipolar disease are more demonstrably emotional even when on an emotionally stable. **(Lebover)**

Just as in Schizophrenia (see section above) there may be some connection to the circadian rhythm of sleep and Bipolar Disease. Afflicted people are often "Night Owls," with delayed sleep cycling timing relative to the rest of us. They are prone to many different sleep disturbances: Insomnia (can't sleep enough), Hypersomnia (too sleepy), and reduced sleep efficiency (waking up a lot and having difficulty going back to sleep).

Frequently, a change in mood is tied to sleep, or lack thereof. **(Lamont)** Sleep deprivation is one of the "on" switches for manic/depressive episodes. So the need for good sleep is critical to disease control. **(Salvadore)** Emotional stability can be severely and adversely affected by irregular sleep patterns. Having a regular nighttime routine with a safe and quiet sleep environment is really important. Staying awake during the day (no naps) helps prepare for sleep in the evening. Medications used to stabilize mood are thought to help synchronize his sleep/wake rhythms as well, so treatment helps support sleep and vice versa. **(Lamont)**

Chapter 16: Normal Aging and Changes in Sleep

"But I have promises to keep, and miles to go before I sleep."
Robert Frost

Like everything else, sleep changes over time. As people age a particular set of issues arise that impact sleep: physical changes, life situations, and illnesses.

Menopause

Q. My wife is going through menopause and is really struggling with sleep, among other things. I realize this is temporary, but what can be done until this phase of her life is over?

Sleep becomes a big issue for many women in their 40s and 50s. Menopause is the transitional stage in a woman's life when her body hormonally and physically loses the ability to naturally get pregnancy. It lasts on average about 4 years all told, beginning with menstrual irregularities and ending with the cessation of periods. While most women welcome not having a period, the process of getting there can be a rough road. For some the change takes as long as a decade. Ten years of fluctuating hormones and physical changes is a long time. And during this episode of a woman's life, sleep can be a real problem.

Perimenopausal women have a variety of sleep complaints. Unsatisfying sleep quality is common due to the myriad problems that arise from hormonal shifts. Hot flashes and sweating are disruptive day and night. Mood shifts and relationship changes also have an impact. Sleeplessness, tiredness and irritability affect professional and personal function. **(Utian)** Good scientific studies demonstrate that perimenopausal women often take longer to get to sleep, wake up more during the night, and sleep less efficiently. **(Kravitz)** Symptom relief can make a big impact.

Hormone replacement therapy (HRT) is a somewhat controversial, but effective, way to minimize hot flashes and moodiness and thereby improve sleep. The controversy stems from the potential risks of estrogen therapy: increased possibilities of endometrial cancer, uterine bleeding, and gallstones. **(Utian)** There is also an increased risk of breast cancer, although the amount of increase is up for debate. If risk factors for breast cancer are already present (like being overweight and having a family history) it may be that HRT should be avoided. Conversely, in the absence of those risk factors it may be okay to start HRT. Some women will choose to be on HRT for a short duration to ease symptoms until they are officially postmenopausal. These are very individual choices and need to be made in consultation with her Gynecologist. **(Chen)**

Hormone replacement therapy has another positive impact from the sleep perspective. Sleep apnea occurs in only about ½% of premenopausal women. Those who are treated with hormone replacement therapy are still pretty unlikely to have OSA, around 1%. Postmenopausal women who are not on HRT have a rate of sleep apnea that approached that of men, around 5%. **(Punjabi)**

Your wife will some day move beyond this phase in her life. A decision about the use of HRT, or not, should be made with her doctor. In the mean time support her, love her, and keep the ceiling fan on.

Normal Aging and Changes in Sleep

Q. I am 82 years old and my kids are giving me the devil about my sleep. They say, "Grandpa, you sleep all day long." Or they complain that I go to bed too early, or get up too early. Why won't they just leave me the hell alone and let me sleep the way I want to? I am doing just fine the way I am!

It is true that sleep changes as we age. There are measurable differences comparing older to younger adults during sleep studies. The elderly have less deep (Stage 3 and REM) sleep and more frequently awaken during the night. It also takes longer to fall asleep. (For a refresher course on sleep and sleep stages, see Chapter 1, What is Sleep?) Often, fewer hours are spent asleep at night, which may explain why the elderly take a lot of naps. They may be the way an old body makes up for the lack of nighttime sleep. **(Edwards)**

The circadian timing of life (see Chapter 7, Circadian Rhythm Disorders for more information) becomes less rigid as we age. Elderly people are frequently in and out of bed earlier than

179

younger folks. **(Neikrug)** Just look at the popularity of the early bird special at Luby's®! There is nothing wrong with this schedule. It is just out of sync with everyone else.

Finally, some sleep diagnoses are more common in older people. Insomnia is frequent. And the use of sedatives to combat it is more common in elderly women than men. **(Edwards)** Sleep Apnea, Restless Legs Syndrome, snoring, and REM Behavior Disorder are all more common in the elderly, particularly men. **(Wolkove)**

However, most of the time, sleep in the elderly is just timed differently and a little less efficient. That doesn't mean that you aren't sleeping well. So I would tell those young whippersnappers to back off and leave the old man alone. If you want to nap, go to bed early, wake up early, and do your own thing, go ahead. You have earned it!

Elder Care Facility/Hospital Sleep

My aging mother is in an assisted living facility and I am not sure how much she is sleeping. I think they do a pretty good job making sure she is in bed safely, but she still seems tired all of the time and complains that her sleep isn't good. What can we do to help her?

A retirement home can be an oasis of care and safety for an elderly person. But, it is sometimes hard to get a good night's sleep in these accommodations. Many aged people live there because they need special care. Physical and mental degradation makes living at home difficult. Arthritic pain limits mobility. Bathing is often difficult. Even getting in and out of bed can be a challenge. Dementia is also common and becoming more so as our society ages. Dementia causes poor sleep, which makes dementia worse. **(Neikrug)** Having help available 24/7 can make a big difference for your mother.

Why is sleep so disrupted in these places? Part of it is the environment in which these folks live. During the day the residents are often inside. Being limited physically due to age and infirmity makes it hard to get out for a walk and some sunshine. There are also many opportunities for naps during the day. Disrupting the waking hours with sleep during the day may lead to disrupted sleep at night. There may also be a lot of nighttime noise and light exposure.

You may say, "So what? She can sleep however shes wants. Leave her alone." And you are correct to a certain degree. But poor sleep has potentially serious negative consequences. People with short sleeping periods at night have a greater risk for falling and shorter survival compared to those who sleep better. **(Martin)**

You can help your mother sleep better at night by keeping her up during the day. Get her outside and exposed to daylight often. Help keep her mind occupied during the daytime so that she stays engaged and alert. Keep nighttime intrusions to a minimum. In other words, she needs good Sleep Hygiene. (See Chapter 2, Advice for Smarter Sleep, page 10 for a more complete discussion of this topic.)

If needed, her doctor can provide a prescription sleeping pill. But, avoid medication if you can. Sedatives can worsen an elderly person's state of mind. Finally, if your mother is depressed, which is not uncommon in the elderly and infirm, counseling and appropriate anti-depressant medication can really help too.

Q. My grandmother is in the ICU and is losing her marbles. They say this is common in older people in the hospital, but she seems to be getting worse. Should I be worried?

Sleep in a hospital setting is difficult for anyone. Being in the ICU makes it even worse. Nurses and doctors come in and out of the room no matter what time of the day or night to provide necessary treatment around the clock. It is great to have the care, but the impact on sleep and mental status can be disastrous.

Hospital Acquired Dementia (A.K.A Sundowning) is common when an elderly person is ill, medicated, and has a disrupted sleep routine. Intensive Care Unit patients are known to have extreme sleep disruption as measured by real time sleep studies. Sleep deprivation in the hospital may very well play a role in the development of ICU delirium. **(Weinhaus)** Daytime and nighttime sleep is disrupted with noise and lights. Sleep comes in bits and pieces throughout the day and night, resulting in confusion and disorientation. Unfortunately, this delirium is associated with

181

worse outcomes. Sedative medications are also implicated, ironically, in disrupting sleep by altering normal sleep patterns in the context of the already disrupted sleep environment. **(Sanders)**

There are some things that the hospital can do to try to prevent the development of ICU delirium. Making sure that your grandmother is awake and connected to the world really helps. Having eyeglasses and hearing aids available keeps her from feeling isolated. Making sure she is moving around, exposed to light, and engaged with her caretakers during daylight hours helps to align sleep and wake schedules with the outside world. Also, having the nursing and medical staff repeatedly engage with her about the time and date helps to keep her oriented. If delirium sets in despite the best efforts of the staff and family, medications typically used to treat psychosis (Haldol® (haloperidol)) are effective at calming her down. **(Girard)** ICU stays are tough for anyone. Make sure you keep in touch with your grandmother while she is in there.

Section 8: Pills and Potions

Chapter 17: Medications and Sleep

Americans use lots of medications. And that is a good thing. The miracles of modern medicines enable us to live longer, healthier lives by treating diseases that were uniformly fatal in our grandparents' generation. We also now have many more treatment options for mental health.

A recommendation to start a new medication comes from your healthcare provider's experience and knowledge of you, your needs, and medical research. No medication is 100% safe or effective. But the alternative of not being treated is often worse. So it is important to weigh the risks, benefits, and alternatives of any suggested treatment. Always ask questions before starting any drug. Get as many answers as you need to make good decisions <u>with</u> your doctor about <u>your</u> health. This is a team sport!

Medications can affect sleep, but only if they are able to enter the brain. Fortunately, this is a very difficult thing to do! Blood vessels in the brain are unique. Using what is called the 'Blood Brain Barrier" they block noxious substances from crossing from the circulation into the body's most critical organ. If a medicine passes through this blockade it may impact brain function. The effect once a drug gets through is the subject of this chapter. We'll go over the most common medications that affect sleep.

One very important note to the reader: the medication effects described are what <u>usually</u> happen to <u>most</u> people. Not everyone has the exact same reaction to a drug. So if your experience is different than the description, neither is wrong.

A key to the tables below is in order before you move on...
- <u>Time to fall asleep</u> = self-explanatory. Quicker indicates a sedative effect.
- <u>Sleep continuity</u> = ability to stay asleep. More (↑)is better than less (↓).
- <u>Slow wave sleep</u> = deep restorative sleep. More (↑) is better than less (↓).
- <u>REM sleep</u> = dream sleep. More (↑)may induce nightmares or may improve restfulness. Less (↓)results in less restful sleep.

-<u>Total sleep time</u> = hours of sleep. More (↑)may indicate a
sedative effect. Less (↓)results in daytime
sleepiness.
(If you need a primer on sleep stages, try reading What is
Sleep? in Chapter 1.)

<u>Alcohol</u>

Drinking to induce sleep is as old as ancient Greece. In fact
Dionysus, the god of pleasure (and having a good time in general) is
credited with this bit of advice…

I mix three drinks for the temperate:
One for health, which they empty first,
The second for love and pleasure,
The third for sleep.
When these cups are emptied, the wise go home.
The fourth drink is ours no longer, but belongs to
violence,
The fifth to uproar,
The sixth to drunken revelry,
The seventh to black eyes,
The eighth to the police,
The ninth to anger,
And the tenth to madness and the hurling of
furniture. **(Dionysus)**

Dionysus was correct that alcohol makes you fall asleep. But
the quality of that sleep is often poor.

Researchers have studied imbibed people to determine how
alcohol impacts sleep. Sounds like tempting research to volunteer
for, doesn't it? The results aren't that rosy, though. Drunken people
fall asleep more quickly than sober ones. And, at least initially, sleep
is really deep. However, any benefit wanes in the early morning
hours. Alcohol affected sleep is characterized by less dream (REM)
sleep and frequent early morning disruptions. Because normal sleep
patterns are not achieved, sleep is less refreshing. **(Arendt)**

Alcoholics are also frequently Insomniacs, using drinks as
sleep aids. Unfortunately, chronic overuse of alcohol is chronically

disruptive to sleep. Fortunately, abstinence from alcohol, or a return to moderate drinking, gets sleep back on track. **(Bower)**

Antidepressants

    Insomnia commonly accompanies Depression and Anxiety. One goal of treatment is a return to more normal sleep patterns. **(Bostwick)** And while this is a common outcome, antidepressant medications themselves may negatively impact sleep.

    These medicines work by changing the balance of chemicals in the brain (serotonin/5HT, norepinephrine/NE, and dopamine/DA to name a few) to improve and stabilize mood. The neurotransmitters are thought to be out of equilibrium in people who are depressed and/or anxious. For the most part the neurotransmitters affected are "wake promoters" in the brain. Changing the impact of these transmitters can impact sleep as well.

    The chart below provides a list of common drugs and their impact on sleep. Balancing the impact on mood versus sleep is the important thing.

    If Depression and Anxiety are improving with drug therapy and you are still sleepy during the day, it may be a medication effect. But, don't overlook other sleep problems. You don't want to miss treating Sleep Apnea, Restless Legs Syndrome, or other problems that may be interfering with your rest. **(Kelly)**

Medications	Sleep Effect
SSRIs – increase serotonin (5HT)	
Celexa® (citalopram)	↓ continuity
Lexapro® (escitalopram)	↓ REM sleep
Luvox® (fluvoxamine)	
Paxil®, Pexeva® (paroxetine)	
Prozac®, Sarafem® (fluoxetine)	
Zoloft® (sertraline)	
SNRIs – increase norepinephrine (NE)	
Cymbalta® (duloxetine)	↓ continuity
Pristiq® (desvenlafaxine)	↓ REM sleep

186

Medications	Sleep Effect
Atypical Antidepressants – increase norepinephrine (NE), serotonin (5HT), and dopamine (DA)	
Oleptro® (trazadone)	↑ continuity ↑ slow wave
Remeron® (mirtazipine)	↑ continuity
Wellbutrin® (bupropion)	↓ continuity ↑ REM

Older Antidepressants – increase norepinephrine (NE) and serotonin (5HT)

Anafranil® (clomipramine)	↑ or ↓ continuity
Elavil® (amitriptyline)	↓ REM
Norpramine® (desimpramine)	
Pamelor® (nortriptyline)	
Silenor® (doxepin)	
Surmontil® (trimipramine)	
Tofranil® (imipramine)	
Vivactil® (proptriptyline)	

Monoamine Oxidase Inhibitors (MAOIs) – increase norepinephrine (NE), serotonin (5HT), and dopamine (DA)

Emsam® (selegine)	↑ REM
Marplan® (isocarboxazid)	
Parnate® (tranylcypromine)	

Antiepileptics

Seizures medications act directly on the brain. As a class, they stabilize and reduce abnormal electrical activity that leads to seizures. Sleepiness is a common side effect of these drugs. Sleepiness is also a common result of poorly controlled seizure activity at night. If you are sleepy on these meds make sure that your treatment is maximized and your seizures are controlled before blaming the treatment and looking to switch to a new one.

Medication	Sleep Effects
Tegretol® (carbamazepine)	↓ time to fall asleep ↑ continuity ↑ deep sleep ↓ REM

Medications	Sleep Effect
Lamictal® (lamotrigine)	↓ deep sleep ↑ REM
Keppra® (levetiracetam)	↑ continuity ↑ deep sleep ↓ REM
Topamax® (topiramate)	↓ time to fall asleep ↑ continuity ↑ deep sleep ↑ continuity
Depakote® (valproic acid)	↓ time to fall asleep
Dilantin® (phenytoin)	↑ continuity ↑ deep sleep ↓ REM

Antipsychotics

Every drug in this category works by increasing levels of the neurotransmitter dopamine (DA) in the brain. The effect is to calm and clarify thought, bringing a person with psychosis back to reality. Every antipsychotic medication is sedating, some more than others and especially the older ones. If taken long enough, most people get used the effect and are no longer so sleepy during the day. If you don't eventually clear the cobwebs, switching medications to a less sedating option may be necessary. **(Muench)**

Medications and Class	Sleep Effects
Typical Antipsychotics	
Haldol® (haloperidol)	↑ continuity
Prolixin® (fluphenazine)	↓ REM
Thorazine® (chlorpromazine)	
Trilafon® (perphenazine)	
Atypical Antipsychotics	
Abilify® (aripiprazole)	↑ continuity
Geodon® (ziprasidone)	↓ REM
Invega® (paliperidone)	
Latuda® (lurasidone)	
Risperidal® (respiradone)	

188

Stimulants

Caffeine

Caffeine is a popular, acceptable, and legal way to try to keep alert and improve performance. It improves wakefulness and vigilance. **(Bonnet)** Caffeine works well and, in appropriate doses, is generally safe.

For most of us, coffee is the delivery method of choice. But not all caffeinated beverages are harmless. "Energy drinks" are very popular, particularly among teens and young adults. The "wings" you get from these drinks mostly comes from the massive amounts of caffeine they contain. One "energy drink" can have as much caffeine as 4 cups of home brewed coffee or 2 cups from Starbucks! And they contain all sorts of stuff beside caffeine, including taurine and other so-called "natural" ingredients. What the "natural" stuff does is a truly a mystery, unless you believe the hype. Needless to say, "energy drinks" are not recommended for consumption by physicians. **(Seifert)**

Caffeine has a significant impact on sleep. Consumption makes it harder to fall asleep and decreases deep sleep stages. It takes about 5 hours for half of the caffeine you consume to leave your body. **(Bonnet)** So a cup of coffee after dinner has an effect deep into the night.

Chronic misuse of caffeine has significant consequences. Because sleep isn't restful, when you awaken from caffeine-disrupted-sleep you feel tired. Your daytime tiredness requires more caffeine to keep you awake. Drinking more caffeinated beverages messes with your sleep. Daytime tiredness continues. More caffeine is required. You get the idea. **(Stradling)**

On the next page is a sampling of caffeinated drinks and their stimulant content. **(Utah) (Informer)**

189

DRINK	CAFFEINE (mg)
ALRI Hypershot	500
Ten Hour Energy Shot	422
5 Hour Energy	200
Red Bull®	200
7 Eleven Energy Shot	80
Mountain Dew®	55
Jolt®	71
Coca Cola® Classic	34
Diet Coke®	46
Dr. Pepper® (regular and diet)	41
Big Red®	38
Barq's® Rootbeer	23
Nestea® Sweet Iced Tea	26
Drip Coffee	115-175
Brewed Coffee	80-135
Espresso	100
Iced Tea	47
Hot Tea	60
Green Tea	15
Hot Cocoa	14
Decaffeinated Coffee	3-4

Amphetamines/Methylphenidate

Stimulant medications are prescribed for two main reasons: 1.) To calm and focus and person with ADD/ADHD and 2.) To stimulate wakefulness in a person who is pathologically sleepy. These are two very different uses. They have been used successfully for both for years, though the risk of abuse is significant.

Someone with ADD/ADHD has difficulty with impulse control, attention, and focus. Contrary to what might be expected, treatment with stimulant medications calms and centers the mind. And they work very well, offering him or her a chance to succeed in conventional academic and professional environments where they might otherwise struggle.

Amphetamines improve wakefulness when given to people with sleepiness due to sleep disorders (see Chapter 13, Narcolepsy and the Hypersomnias, for more info) or medical problems (see Chapter 14, strokes, brain injuries, Parkinson's, Multiple Sclerosis). **(Sonka)** Much like caffeine, stimulants also improve vigilance after sleep deprivation. **(Bonnet)** But because of their side effects, and because safer alternative medications are now available, amphetamines are used less frequently, now.

No matter the reason for taking them, when stimulants are taken is important to prevent sleep side effects. Taken too late in the day, stimulants keep you awake and disrupt sleep continuity. Most of the time the last dose should be taken no later then noon so that it is out of the system when it is time for bed.

Tragically, ADD/ADHD meds are commonly abused as recreational drugs. It is estimated that up to 4.1 million people over the age of 12 have used stimulant medication without a prescription. College students are the most likely culprits. **(Arria)** When used illicitly, these medications create euphoria, increased energy, alertness, decreased fatigue, and decreased appetite. Amphetamines are also abused to try to improve academic performance, with mixed results. Some people, generally those who aren't performing well to start with, have very minor improvements in creative thinking, memory, and mental process control. **(Lakhan)** Most who take these drugs don't have much benefit.

In addition to being addictive, there is a nasty side to stimulant abuse: aggressive behavior, hostility, paranoia, headache, nausea, racing heart, convulsions, and hallucinations. Just like other illicit drugs, stopping stimulants after prolonged abuse can lead to withdrawal symptoms. Not a pretty sight.

Illicit use of stimulant medications also results in sleep disruption. Difficulty falling asleep and frequent awakenings during the night **(Bonnet)** causes ineffective rest, daytime sleepiness, and ongoing stimulant abuse. The cycle is a bad one.

Medications	Sleep Effects
Adderal® (amphetamine-dextro amphetamine)	↓ total sleep time ↓ REM
Concerta®,Ritalin® (methylphenidate)	
Dexedrine®, (dextroamphetamine)	

191

Wakefulness Promoters

Provigil® (modafinil) and Nuvigil® (armodafinil) are safer alternatives to amphetamines for people who are too sleepy and need help staying awake. These drugs do not provide the same sort of "high" as the amphetamines, decreasing abuse potential. (Jasinski) Because they lack intense stimulation, wake promoters are not effective in, and therefore not prescribed for, ADD/ADHD. (Wilens)

Provigil® (modafinil) and Nuvigil® (armodafinil) are best used for people who have effectively treated sleep disorders who still have excessive daytime sleepiness. For example, these meds work well for a person with Sleep Apnea who remains sleepy despite objective evidence that the apneas are abolished with CPAP. Shift workers have improved alertness and productivity with them. They are also effective helping people with Narcolepsy combat their daytime drowsiness. (Bonnet)

Like with any stimulant, there are potential side effects. Anxiety, insomnia, loss of appetite, and headaches occur rarely. (Schwarz). The last dose of modafinil/armodafinil should be taken at latest by noon, allowing its wake promotion to wane by bedtime. If timed correctly, there is no adverse affect on sleep stages. (Roth)

Medication	Sleep Effects
Nuvigil® (armodafinil) Provigil® (modafinil)	No impact if taken before noon

Nicotine products

Nicotine delivery systems have multiplied in recent years. You can still go old school and smoke or chew tobacco to get the drug. Smoking cessation tools provide nicotine by chewing gum, nasal sprays, and skin patches. Now, we even have people "vaping" with e-cigarettes, inhaling water vapor laced with nicotine in an imitation of smoking. No matter how that nicotine gets into the system, it can have a negative impact on sleep.

Smokers have a harder time falling asleep, sleep less, and have less deep stage sleep. (Zhang) People who smoke are also more likely to have insomnia. (Fernandez-Mendoza)

Bottom line: Don't smoke, be healthier, and sleep better.

Medication	Sleep Effects
Nicotine	↑ time to fall asleep
	↓ total sleep time
	↓ deep sleep

Pain medicines

Narcotics

"Narco" is derived from a Greek word meaning "stupor" or "numbness." Narcotics do a good job of both.

Short duration narcotic pain relief medications are often prescribed for acute pain after injury or surgery. They include Astramorph® (morphine), Demerol® (meperidine), Tylenol #2/#3/#4/codeine, Norco®/Vicodin® (hydrocodone/tylenol), Percocet® (oxycodone), and Ultram® (tramadol). Each is subtly different from the next one, but all achieve some measure of pain relief. Sleep while taking narcotics is not normal, but it is better than not sleeping due to pain. And when you are healing, sleep is very important.

Many people have chronic pain. They need chronic pain relief. Long-acting medications, like Oxycontin® (extended release oxycodone), Duragesic® (fentanyl patch) , and Methadose® (methadone), provide excellent long-term relief and improve quality of life and productivity. There is an impact on sleep, but without pain relief sleep would be hard to come by. So, take the good with the bad. If you are unlucky enough to need long term, slow release narcotics for pain, use them wisely and carefully.

The price to pay for pain relief can be an expensive one when it comes to sleep. At high enough dosages, narcotics decrease your drive to breath. Sleep Apnea, both Central (Chapter 6) and Obstructive (Chapter 5), is common. **(Farney)** Sleep architecture is also affected. Narcotized sleep has less REM sleep and more deep sleep stages. **(Dimsdale)**

Like all therapies, there are risks and benefits. Be careful with these medications.

Medication	Sleep Effects
Demerol® (meperidine)	↓ total sleep time
Duragesic® (fentanyl)	↓ REM
Oxycontin® (oxycodone controlled release)	↑ deep sleep
Percocet®, Roxicet® (oxycodone)	
Tylenol #3 (codeine)	
Vicodin®/Norco® (hydrocodone)	
Methadose® (methadone)	
Astramorph® (morphine)	

Pain/Seizure Medications

Gabapentin (Neurontin®) and pregabalin (Lyrica®) provide relief from chronic pain without abuse and addiction potential. Both were developed initially for the treatment of seizures but have greater utility in the treatment of pain, particularly that arising from fibromyalgia, nerve inflammation, other neurological pain disorders. They are a Godsend for a lot of people. Both Neurontin® (gabapentin) and Lyrica® (pregabalin) have some miraculous sleep side effects: they actually INCREASE deep (slow wave) sleep, help people fall asleep faster, and stay asleep. **(Roehrs) (Boomershine)**

Medication	Sleep Effects
Neurontin® (gabapentin)	↓ time to fall asleep
Lyrica® (pregabalin)	↑ slow wave sleep
	↑ sleep continuity

Sleeping pills

In 2010 there were 108 million prescriptions filled for sedative medications. **(IMS)** It is estimated that 4% of American adults use sleep medications. **(Chong)** That's a lot of people who need help going to sleep!

There are a lot of sleeping pills out there to choose from, both OTC and prescription. Obviously any pill that is supposed to help you sleep is going to have an impact on sleep, which is both the problem and the desired effect with all of them. They absolutely help you fall and stay asleep. But sedative induced sleep is not for the most party normal. Sleep stages and restfulness are often affected. Trying to strike a balance is key. It is better to sleep unmedicated. However, Chronic Insomnia is much worse than any negative sleep impact due to a pill.

The most popular prescribed sleeping pills are Ambien® (zolpidem), Ambien CR® (zolpidem tartrate) and Lunesta® (eszopiclone) – the so-called "Z" drugs. These are newer and safer relatives of the Valium® (diazepam) family of drugs, that are also commonly prescribed for sleep. **(Pagel)**

Any drug that makes you sleepy can be used for a sedative. And while they are not intended to be used for sleep, Oleptro® (trazodone) and Elavil®(amitriptyline) are the two most popular prescriptions in this category. Because they are antidepressants, they may improve mood disorders and sleep at the same time. Between these two, primary care physicians wrote almost 10 million prescriptions for sleep in 2006. **(Lai)** (See the Antidepressant list above for information on how they affect sleep.)

A newer drug, Rozerem® (ramelteon) has a very different mechanism of action. It does not actively sedate. It acts similarly to Melatonin, binding on the receptors that help to initiate the onset of sleep. **(Neubauer)** It seems to be effective without causing drowsiness, particularly in Alzheimer's Disease.

The newest drug is Belsomra® (suvorexant). It has a novel approach to putting you to sleep. It is the first medication that inhibits the action of orexin, a brain chemical that stimulates wakefulness. So it doesn't make you sleepy, it keeps you from being awake. **(Sun)**

There are also effective over-the-counter sleep aids. The older antihistamines Benadryl® (diphenhydramine) and Unisom® (doxylamine) make you extremely sleepy. **(Adam)** But, just because a medicine is over the counter doesn't mean that it is side effect free. Be careful with any medication you take to help you sleep, regardless of where you got it.

A final word on these medications: never mix sedatives. They can be dangerous if not used correctly. And never drink alcohol or take any other recreational drug with your sleeping pill. The combined effects can be deadly. Be safe and careful with any and all medication.

Medication	Sleep Effects
"Z" Drugs	
Ambien® (zolpidem)	↓ time to fall asleep
Ambein CR® (zolpidem Tartrate)	No sleep stage changes
Lunesta® (eszopiclone)	↓ time to fall asleep Occasional hangover
Benzodiazepines	
Ativan® (lorazepam)	↓ time to fall asleep
Halcion® (triazolam)	↓ REM
Klonopin® (clonazepam)	
Restoril® (temazepam)	
Valium® (diazepam)	
Xanax® (alprazolam)	
Melatonin Agonist	
Rozerem® (ramelteon)	No sleep stage changes
Orexin Inhibitor	
Belsomra® (suvorexant)	↓ time to fall asleep ↑ continuity
Anti-histamines	
Benadryl® (diphen-hydramine)	↑ stage 2 sleep ↓ REM
Unisom® (doxylamine)	

Medications for Restless Legs Syndrome (RLS)

Any medication that affects brain chemistry is bound to have some effect on sleep. RLS treatment includes medications that stimulate dopamine brain receptors. Fortunately they help people with RLS fall asleep. **(Ferreira)** Some effect on sleep stages and sedation is common.

Medication	Sleep Effects
Dopamine Enhancer	
Requip® (ropinirole)	Vivid dreams ↓ time to fall asleep ↓ REM ↑ continuity

Medication	Sleep Effects
Dopmine Enhancer	
Mirapex® (pramipexole)	Sedating
	↓ time to fall asleep
	↑ continuity
Anti-epileptics	
Neurontin® (gabapentin) and	↓ time to fall asleep
Lyrica® (pregabalin)	↑ slow wave sleep
	↑ sleep continuity

Heart rhythm and blood pressure medications

Cardiovascular medications, perhaps surprisingly, may affect sleep if they cross over into the brain.

Anti-arrhythmics (medications for irregular heat beats) often have sedation side effects. With continued usage most people become accustomed to the effect and are no longer so sleepy.

Some medications for high blood pressure have an impact on sleep beyond drowsiness. A few of the beta blockers (like Inderal®(propranolol)) have an effect at serotonin (5HT) receptors as well with really bizarre results for some people. Not only do they occasionally cause sleepiness, but they can also stimulate very intense dreams and even nightmares. This effect can get bad enough to necessitate a change to a different treatment. **(Neubauer)** Catapres® (clonidine), which is an "alpha 2 blocker" can have a similar effect, causing significant sedation and nightmares.

Minipress® (prazosin), an "alpha 1 blocker," has quite the opposite effect. It decreases REM sleep and decreases nightmares. Minipress® (prazosin) is used successfully for Post Traumatic Stress Disorder (PTSD) and Nightmare Disorder. **(Aurora)**

Medication	Sleep Effects
Antiarrythmics	
Betapace® (sotalol)	↓ continuity
	insomnia
	nightmares/vivid dreams
Beta Blockers	
Inderal® (propranolol)	↓ continuity
Lopressor® (metoprolol)	↓ REM

Medication	Sleep Effects
Beta Blockers	
Visken®(pindolol)	nightmares
Alpha Blockers	
Catapres® (clonidine)	↑ deep sleep
	↓ REM
	nightmares
Minipress® (prazosin)	↑ deep sleep
	↓ REM
	relief from nightmares

Asthma medications

Asthmatics often have more wheezing at night, so their sleep suffers. (See Chapter 14, Medical Problems and Sleep.) So treating asthma improves sleep. However, the very medications that decrease nighttime wheezing sometimes interfere with a good night's sleep.

Asthma medications dilate the airways in the lungs to treat/prevent wheezing. Inhaled short acting medicines, like Proair® (albuterol), and long acting drugs, like Advair® (salmeterol-fluticasone) work by stimulating adrenalin receptors. Wheezing is treated or prevented by the relaxation of small airway tubules in the lungs called bronchioles.

Some of that inhaled medicine makes its way through the lungs and is absorbed into the bloodstream. If it makes it all the way to the brain, adrenalin receptors are stimulated and sleep can be disturbed.

Other older medications, like Uniphyl® (aminophylline) and Theodur® (theophylline), are taken in pill form to relax bronchioles and prevent wheezing. They act in the brain very similarly to caffeine, blocking brain fatigue and stimulating wakefulness.

Finally, anti-inflammatory steroids, which decrease lung inflammation and reactivity, are useful for asthmatics. Their impact on sleep is discussed below.

An asthmatic with good control of their wheezing that isn't sleeping well should talk to their doctor about their treatment. **(Welsh)** Adjusting the timing, dosages, and/or changing medications may be necessary.

Medication	Sleep Effects
Broncho®ilators	
Proair® (albuterol)	Insomnia if taken close too
Advair® (salmeterol/ Fluticasone)	close to bedtime
Oral Asthma Medications	
Uniphyl® (aminophylline)	↓ continuity
Theodur® (theophylline)	↓ slow wave sleep insomnia

Allergy medications

Antihistamines are notorious for causing drowsiness. Since histamine is one of the chemicals in the brain that promotes wakefulness, blocking it with an "anti" histamine will make you long for a nap. **(Proctor)** The older class of medications that includes Benadryl® (diphenhydramine), Chlortrimeton® (chlorpheniramine), and Tavist® (clemastine) have this side effect so potently that some people use them for sleep aids. Newer over-the-counter allergy medications, like Allerga® (fexofenadine), Zyrtec® (cetirizine) and Claritin® (loratidine) are available. Because they don't readily cross the blood brain barrier they don't cause drowsiness.

The use of anti-inflammatory steroids is common in the treatment of allergy flares acutely. For more information, see the next section.

Medication	Sleep Effects
Benadryl®(diphen-hydramine)	↑ stage 2 sleep ↓ REM
ChlorTrimeton® (chlor-pheniramine)	
Tavist® (clemastine)	
Allegra® (fexofenadine)	No effect on sleep
Claritin® (loratidine)	
Zyrtec® (cetirizine)	

Corticosteriods

Anti-inflammatory steroids are double-edged swords. They are life saving when treating chronic severe asthma and autoimmune diseases (like Lupus and Rheumatoid Arthritis). Without the steroids these conditions are often fatal.

Side effects of prolonged steroid use for these diseases are widespread and severe: weight gain, adrenal gland problems, high blood pressure, diabetes, and cataracts, among others. Most of the time, when faced with a life threatening illness, accepting the side effects in exchange for improved quality and quantity of life is worth it.

Steroids are also used in short bursts for less life threatening problems: severe allergic reactions, asthma flare-ups, and some infections. Side effects still occur, but aren't so dire. Short-term use of steroids can provide a sense of energy and disrupt sleep. Putting up with some hyperactivity and poor sleep to fix a more significant medical problem is reasonable. Just be aware that if your doctor prescribes steroids you may be in for some sleepless nights. **(Schweitzer)**

Medication	Sleep Effects
Decadron® (dexamethasone)	↓ continuity
Deltasone® (prednisone)	↓ slow wave sleep
Solucortef® (hydrocortisone)	↓ REM
Medrol® (methylprednisolone)	

Chapter 18: Complementary and Alternative Medicines (CAM) and Treatments

"Sleep is the best meditation."
Dalai Lama

Many people are reluctant to discuss their use of herbs and folk medicine with doctors. And to be fair, many doctors are not at all accepting of anything not included in the medical school curriculum. It is difficult for doctors to stray from the science of sleep and medicine.

On the one hand I am all for effective, safe treatments, no matter where they come from. On the other hand as a physician I am extremely hesitant to recommend things that have not been explored with scientific rigor, especially if they have the potential to cause harm. We weigh risks and benefits whenever prescribing any therapy in medicine. I cannot weigh what I don't know – and that is where you find the majority of the complementary and alternative approaches. If an alternative treatment is carefully evaluated and found to be effective, with benefits that outweigh risks, it becomes mainstream. For example, Melatonin was initially an alternative therapy. Real sleep medicine research took it off the CAM list and landed it in the doctor's office. But, if a complementary therapy is tested and seen to be ineffective, I find it hard to suggest its use.

One other thing on the topic of traditional western medicine versus alternative treatments; just because it is purported to be "natural" doesn't mean it is harmless or even safe. Opium and arsenic are very natural substances. I don't think anyone believes that they are harmless. Think carefully about taking something we don't know much about. "Popping pills" from the pharmacy is somehow deemed to be more dangerous than popping a handful of supplement tablets from the whole-earth-fair-trade-free-range-organic-natural-pill bottle. As a doctor, I am always skeptical of any therapy until it has proven its worth. As a health consumer, I would suggest you do the same.

Some of what is listed below is quackery. But I will try to point out things that are helpful (or at least not harmful) for your consideration.

201

Insomnia and CAM

According to the National Institute for Health 1.4% of Insomniacs surveyed have tried some CAM to help them sleep, most of which were herbal remedies. Almost 40% of them also tried relaxations techniques. **(NIH1)** That says to me that an Insomniac is trying really hard to get a good night's sleep. And can you blame them?

The supplement aisle is packed with sleep aids. Unfortunately most are not better than a sugar pill (placebo) when put to the scientific test. Relaxation techniques, on the other hand, can make a big difference. Read on to hear about the science.

Herbal Supplements

Chamomile

A really good randomized, blinded, comparative trial was performed pitting chamomile extract in pill form versus a placebo pill. There was no measureable effect. There were two noteworthy findings, though. First, people with placebo slept longer than those on chamomile. Second, people on placebo had more side effects. While there seems to be very little downside to drinking chamomile tea, it doesn't make you sleepy. **(Zick)**

Valerian

This herbal supplement is derived from the root of a plant by the same name and is said to induce sleepiness. In one particularly good study Valerian was put to the test in a group of older women who had trouble sleeping. The research subjects did not know if they were on a standardized dose of valerian (from a supplement company) or a placebo (sugar pill). The women were subjected to all sorts of measurements to gauge any effect. They were asked about the quality of their sleep and their lives. Their sleep was also studied in a sleep lab.

There were no differences in self-reported or scientifically obtained sleep measures between the 2 groups. Also, of note, there were no reported side effects from either group. **(Taibi)** Meh. No upside, no downside.

L-tryptophan

This is an amino acid that is famously present in turkey and blamed for naps after Thanksgiving dinner. L-tryptophan supplements are sold to try to recreate that post-feast feeling and help people fall asleep. The good news is that it does seem to have some positive impact if taken at the right dose. **(George)** However, L-tryptophan has a bit of a checkered history.

Eosinophilia-myalgia syndrome (EMS) is as awful as it sounds. Disabling, severe muscle pains, scarring of the skin and internal organs, and inflammation of the muscle coverings (fascia) characterize the syndrome. **(NIH1)** There was an outbreak of EMS in 1989. At the time there was no known cause, though it was always associated with the use of L-tryptophan. **(Allen) (Tagaki)** By the mid 90's L-tryptophan was taken off the shelves. It was determined that a source for the supplement had a contaminant that may have caused EMS. Since it was reintroduced in 2005 there have been very few cases. That said, I can't recommend L-tryptophan. The risk, though small, outweighs any benefit, which is also small.

Kava

This is another dietary supplement that has problems. It is from the South Pacific, so what could go wrong, right? Well it doesn't seem to help you sleep well. **(NIH1)** And there is this little thing about a warning issued by the FDA about potential liver injury. **(Ringdahl)**

Kava doesn't work. And it can harm you. Stay away.

Energy Meridians and Relaxation Techniques

Relaxation helps you sleep. And relaxing is a prime focus of Traditional Asian Medicine (TAM), which is great. But for some reason, though, most of you who practice TAM don't let your Western medical doctor know about it. **(Bertisch)** Part of that may be our fault as physicians. The attitudes of most MDs toward these approaches to health usually range from dismissive to grudging acceptance. But it does help us care for you as a whole person if we know all about you. And, some of these methods are scientifically tested and seem to be effective. **(Kozasa)** So you should share if it helps with your healthcare.

For a Sleep Medicine physician to recommend any therapy there has to be some scientific proof. And, yes, it is true that Western techniques are not always scientifically valid. But, on the whole, we do try to figure out whether a treatment is warranted based on the scientific method. Personally, I would not want my doctor thinking any other way.

A lot of you search for an alternative path to a good night of sleep. Good for you. From my perspective, as long as something doesn't harm you, and you don't turn your back on proven therapies, why not give it a try?

Let's go through some of these non-medical approaches to Insomnia that really seem to make a difference.

Energy Meridians: Acupressure, Shiatsu, Acupuncture, and Electroacupuncture

These techniques are grounded in traditional Chinese medicine so western scientific literature about them is sparse. But there are studies that demonstrate scientifically valid improvement in sleep using these approaches.

Acupressure focuses on about 150 pressure points on meridians of the body. Manipulation of these points is intended to balance energy and improve health. Scientific evaluation of acupressure has found some benefits for sleep quality. One good study assessed a wristband acupressure device that influenced the "Shen Men" point on the wrist. Sleep studies were performed with or without the bracelet. They showed improvement in a lot of the things you want to see: better sleep efficiency, shorter time to fall asleep, and more total time asleep. **(Carotenuto)** Verifying this with additional studies will add credibility to this treatment.

Shiatsu uses the same meridians and pressure points as acupressure but also provides a whole body massage. Unfortunately, it has not been studied as much. Results are mixed for Shiatsu and sleep in rigorous scientific studies. Those that have been done were fairly inconclusive with no demonstrable benefits. **(Robinson)**

Acupuncture manipulates the meridian energy field with

needles instead of pressure or massage. There is a relative lack of good science measuring this practice in sleep. However a review of the limited scientific literature shows that it may provide some improvement. We can't know for sure until it has been tested for real with scientific rigor. Acupuncture seems to be relatively safe thought, so there is very little downside. **(Cao)**

Electroacupuncture uses the same acupuncture approach to the traditional Chinese medicine meridian sites. A very low voltage electric current is added to the needles to enhance the effect. A randomized, controlled study was performed on electroacupuncture. And while it was a small group of patients, there was some interesting data. Compared to people who had sham acupuncture, the "electrified" ones had better sleep both by report and by measurement. There were few if any complications in the treatment group related to the needles. **(Yeung)**

If you are an adherent to traditional Chinese medicine, and you are having trouble sleeping, some of these techniques may benefit you. There is certainly no downside. As more information becomes available through good scientific study I hope that we will find more safe and effective non-medical approaches.

Relaxation Techniques: Tai Chi, Yoga, and Meditation

Sticking with the Far Eastern arts, we turn to Tai Chi Chih which is described as a slow moving meditation. Starting as a martial art/self-defense technique in ancient China, "tai chi" is interpreted as "supreme ultimate fist!" From there it has evolved into a form of exercise and relaxation to improve health. It is particularly effective for older adults as an excellent form of gentle and graceful exercise and meditation. **(NIH2)** Both of those things help sleep, for certain. But what does the science say?

One study looked at people who had mild sleep complaints but did not have chronic Insomnia. Participants who learned Tai Chi did much better than those who only received sleep education. **(Irwin)** Something so safe and helpful as Tai Chi is easy to recommend. It is a very nice way to relax, stretch, and get some exercise, all of which are helpful for sleep. Give it a try.

205

Yoga is an ancient physical and spiritual practice. It uses very specific postures and meditations intended to still internal dissonance and turmoil. The harmonizing of mind and body to a placid and centered peaceful state is the ultimate goal. That is ideal from a sleep perspective.

When evaluated scientifically, yoga is helpful for people with some medical problems. Cancer patients successfully use yoga to lower stress and improve sleep. **(Cohen)** Women with osteoarthritis feel better and have better self reported sleep quality with yoga practice. **(Taibi)** There is no scientific information yet about chronic Insomnia and yoga. But here again we have an approach to sleep improvement that has little downside. The relaxation and physical improvement that yoga provides can only benefit sleep. So it is worth a try.

Meditation involves the alteration of one's mind until all thought and mental activity is extinguished except for a pure state of awareness of self. Wow. That is deep. So what does that have to do with sleep? Actually quite a bit.

There was a great study done looking at sleep study data from long-term meditators compared to people who had not achieved such consciousness. Practitioners described experiencing "witnessing sleep" during which the meditator is a peaceful inner observer of awaking, sleeping and dreaming. Compared to non-meditators, these people have demonstrably different sleep during a sleep study. They had less muscle tone in deep sleep and much more intense dream sleep (REM) cycles. They also had an unusual combination of deep sleep and waking brain wave patterns, supporting their contention that they are aware of these typically unconscious states. **(Mason)** What does that mean for someone with Insomnia? I can't say. But the impact on sleep is real, so there may be hope. As of now, there aren't any studies looking at meditation as a stand-alone treatment for Insomnia as compared to counseling, medications, or other interventions. (You can read all about these in Chapter 3, Insomnia.) It is a reasonable addition to non-medical Insomnia care, though. Hopefully we will soon find confirmation this promising technique.

As with many of these relaxation techniques, meditation is

completely harmless. If you are good at it and meditation helps, knock yourself out!

Chapter 19: Crazy Quackery and Sleep

"The practice of physic (Medicine) is jostled by quacks on the one
side, and by science on the other."
Peter Mere Latham

Millions of people have difficulty sleeping due to Insomnia
or Sleep Apnea or Restless Legs or Sleep Walking/Talking or....you
name it. Wherever there is a medical problem you can usually find
somebody devising and advertising a guaranteed remedy, trying to
score a little income on an unsuspecting and ill informed public.
Snake oil cures have been around forever.

One of the goals of this book is to dispel myths and educate
about sleep. A person armed with knowledge can advocate for him
or herself. Use science as your guide.

We now venture away from such high-minded pursuits to
delve into the world of fakery and sham cures. Be aware, lots of
people fall for these. If you have found yourself tempted to try
something that sounded too good to be true, remember that the old
saying is correct. Rarely is there a single pill, maneuver, or throat
spray that is going to magically make ANYTHING get better. Be
very skeptical. And if you have questions, ask your doctor.

You need to know one thing before reading what follows:
none of these actually work to cure whatever it is they propose to
cure.

Snoring and Sleep Apnea

Snoring is such a common problem that there are an
abundance of maneuvers and devices and sprays and supplements
that supposedly makes it all stop. If only it was this easy…

-EXERCISES - That Don't Work to Stop Snoring and Apnea

Gimmicky maneuvers intended to "improve the strength and
tone" of the throat keeping it open to quiet snoring/Sleep Apnea.

- Yawn repeatedly
- Sing for 20-30 minutes a day

208

- Stick the tip of the tongue into the back of the mouth
- Open your mouth as widely as possible and hold it there repeatedly
- Say "The lips, the teeth, the tip of the tongue" over and over.
- Stick the tongue out of the mouth as far as you can and move it side to side without touching the corners of the mouth
- Pretend to blow a kiss
- Pretend to suck up juice (not milk for some reason) as if through a straw
- Exaggerated movements of the face and mouth to exercise the muscles
- Push the jaw out and hold it there
- Hold a pencil in the mouth (to strengthen jaw muscles)

Does it hurt to do mouth, face and throat exercises? Nope. Do those exercises cure snoring and sleep apnea? Of course not.

-FOODS - That Don't Help Stop Snoring and Apnea

Some foods are said to "reduce airway congestion" and decrease snoring. I am a bit skeptical that expensive shellfish make that much of a difference. Check out the list:

- Oranges, lemons, and grapefruit – citrus in general
- Onions, garlic, and leeks. (Seems to me that they would just result in your sleeping alone due to bad breath – thus no complaints about your snoring!)
- Lobster – oh I wish I had a bad snoring problem so I could try this one out
- Substituting fish for red meat
- Mustard and thyme
- Pears
- Horseradish

And of course there are foods that supposedly <u>cause</u> snoring and NEED to be avoided! Most of these are high in calories, which does tend to increase girth and, with it, snoring. However, Velveeta® supposedly has some direct effect on the throat. There you have it, mac and cheese causes snoring...

- Cheese food (like Velveeta® - no queso for you!)
- Dairy
- Eggs
- Wheat and corn
- Sugar
- Baked goods (sorry Girl Scouts)
- And of course refined oils and fats

-DIETARY SUPPLEMENTS - That Do Nothing to Stop Snoring and Apnea

No surprise that there are supplements marketed to help you stop snoring. There are supplements that are supposed to help with just about everything. Are any of them tested scientifically? Not many. If they were tested and determined to be ineffective the market for the product might disappear. There are plenty of misguided and good-hearted people who sell these "natural" products that they <u>just know</u> can help.

Natural is not always harmless though. The main problem with these products is lack of information. The Food and Drug Agency considers supplements to be foods, not the drugs that they are. So there is little regulation and no requirement for real scientific safety and effectiveness testing. So they may not work and, what's worse, they may not be safe. That is why there are disclaimers like this one on all of these products: "These products are intended to support general wellbeing and are not intended to treat, diagnose, mitigate, prevent, or cure any condition or disease. If conditions persist, please seek advice from your medical doctor."

Despite that warning, people still pin their hopes to them.

- Snore formula pills. These usually contain a variety of herbs, digestive enzymes, and amino acids. Lots of the homeopathic

210

ones contain "Nux Vomicum." Tasty! The ones from Asia often don't even tell you what is in them. Most of them say that they decrease the amount of mucous that accumulates in the back of the throat opening the airway to make snoring disappear. If only it were that easy.

- Throat and nose sprays. Most of these have some form of menthol or mint, maybe some glycerin and a little alcohol. The idea is to lubricate the throat so that it doesn't vibrate while you are asleep. I have had more than one patient in the office that sheepishly admitted that they fell for this ruse. No, they don't work.
- Snore strips. These are like small breath mint strips that contain essential oils and vitamins that "lubricate" the back of the throat and tongue to prevent the snoring vibration. Same answer – doesn't work.

-SNORING DEVICES - That Are A Waste Of Money for Treatment of Snoring and Apnea

Occasionally desperate times call for desperate measures. And if you are on the cusp of being kicked out of the bedroom to the couch in the basement, a trial of one of these devices doesn't look too bad. There are bunches of them. Some look pretty uncomfortable. Unfortunately, none of the things listed here work. Really. I wish I know who came up with all of this stuff.

- Snore relief nasal ring magnets. This device, which when worn looks as if you are part of a psychedelic tribe of Bornean jungle dwellers, sits in your nostrils while you sleep. The magnets supposedly stimulate sensory nerves in the nose that open the nasal passage. It may stop snoring, the marketing pitch says. Always hedge your bets when selling snake oil.
- Nose dilators. These plastic or silicon cones fit up into the nostrils to help keep the nose open. Some of these have very specific claims – 84% relief of snoring and sleep apnea. Not sure where they obtained their data, because of course they don't say. Some also claim to decrease blood pressure and infections.

211

- Chin straps. These are bands of elastic material that you wear around your head to keep you mouth shut when you sleep. They supposedly retrain your mouth and throat to return to normal and help you stop snoring.
- Didgeridoo. That's right. The Australian aboriginal musical instrument. Its consistent use is supposed to improve the muscle tone of the airway and reduce Sleep Apnea. Amazingly, there is a Swiss study that reported improved sleep study results comparing didgeridoo playing versus doing nothing. In the study both groups had decreased sleep apnea severity after 4 months. **(Puhan)** And the didgeridoo group improved slightly, and statistically meaningfully, more than the group that did nothing. The part that they didn't discuss is that all of the participants still had sleep apnea! Give me something that is less noisy and works.
- Electric shock wristbands. These devices apply a small amount of current every time it hears a snore, supposedly training the wearer to learn to sleep in a position that does not stimulate snoring. It is described in one ad as a biofeedback device, which I guess is true.
- Reminder message device. This is a "revolutionary" new way to stop snoring. You wear an earpiece that is connected to a sound activated digital message. When you snore you hear something like, "Hey, turn over." Better than an elbow I guess.

-INSOMNIA CURES - That Cure Nothing

There are bunches of "medical devices" available to help someone get a good night's sleep without medication. I am all for that. Unfortunately, the ads suggest that all you have to do is use this machine/device to get good sleep. Forget about relaxation and good Sleep Hygiene. Another magic cure. Entertaining, yes. Helpful, no.

- Negative ion therapy. You heard it right. This is a Chinese "medicine" approach. Somehow when the device is attached to the body it streams negative ions that are supposed to cure everything from hay fever to

Insomnia. They even claim it improves immune function. Wow. It's on the Internet so it must be true.

- Electrical waveforms. This approach comes in many forms and brand names. Basically electrical current "waveforms" are applied to the scalp. This energy reportedly gets into the brain to regulate levels of brain chemicals. The current is too weak to be noticed so it doesn't even hurt! Of course it has to be used for a long period of time. But persistence pays off. Anxiety, Depression, and Insomnia are cured with this simple application. "Research" (which is murkily presented) "proves" the results. They claim up to 90% of their "clients" have relief. Some even claim to instill a sense of optimism. Pretty amazing stuff, but too good to be true.
- Brain freeze! Believe it or not, a patent was granted for a device that cools the forehead – er, um I mean uses hypothermia of the frontal lobe of the brain – to treat Insomnia. I am sure that if it ever makes it to market it will be really expensive. Maybe eating a snow cone could be a cheaper alternative?
- Electroacupressure. At least that is what it seems to be to me. These devices, at least four of which must be bought and worn for effect, are placed on the wrists and the feet. An undetectable electrical current, I assume similar to electroacupuncture, is applied to these points. The electricity supposedly affects the energy meridian to improve an amazing amount of problems: anxiety, nausea, indigestion, and irritability. And as an added bonus even chronic and severe insomniacs get sleep relief. Of course something this amazing comes at a price – a pretty steep one.
- Light machine. This one is genius. You turn it on when you are trying to go to sleep. As the light brightness undulates you are supposed to match your breathing to its rhythm. As time goes on it slows the pace of your breathing. After a short period of time the light shuts off and you roll over and go to sleep. Not only do they claim that relaxation ensues, this product supposedly reduces cortisol, which they say improves melatonin production.

213

Not sure who came up with this one but they must make a killing based on the cost of the lights versus the level of technology.

- The handheld Insomnia computer. This apparatus not only monitors your sleep, it gives you feedback and tells you how to cure your Insomnia. The computer does a lot of work to help you out. During the first week it learns about your sleep patterns. It determines if you are asleep by seeing if you wake up to a noise. (I am not making this up.) Once it sees your sleeping pattern it makes recommendations about when to go to sleep and when to get up. Really. Once you are trained, continued use maintains your now excellent sleep. Good luck with that.

There are many more of these out there. Let the buyer beware.

Section 9: The Technical Discussion

"You can't handle the truth."
Col. Jessep, A Few Good Men.

Chapter 20: The Science of Sleep 101

Welcome. You have come to the back of the book...the part they warned you about. The nerdy place where those who NEED to know come to get the science. You will have a much richer understanding of this book by having read this section. Don't worry. I won't tell anyone. I'm actually proud that you are willing to delve into this greater detail. I think you will be glad you did.

What follows is my attempt to interpret some very complicated and not yet well-understood science to someone who isn't a physician or a researcher. There are a lot of things we know about sleep and a lot more we don't. I will give you the latest version of what we understand that relates to the content of this book. I will try my best not to bore you or fill these pages with unnecessary details that don't help your comprehension of sleep and its problems. If the information changes I will be sure to update this section in future editions.

There is no test (at least for you - I had to take one!) No need to regurgitate this for an oral presentation, I promise. In fact this stuff isn't even necessary to get what you need out of this book. But, I want to present this to you in case you were one of those people who needed to know the "why" and not just the "what." That said...here we go...

The Brain

Before we can have a discussion of the science of sleep, some basic information about the function and structure of the brain is in order. Completely understanding the brain is pretty much impossible even for brain scientists, at least at this point in time. But research has discovered some of how the brain works and what happens when parts aren't working well. Part of that understanding has led to insights into what controls sleep and waking.

The brain is made up of more than 100 million nerve cells (neurons). They are intricately interconnected and communicate in ways more complicated than we can currently imagine. Each cell-to-cell communication generates a small amount of electricity. Those bits of energy created by so many interacting neurons add up, so much so that we can detect them with sensors on the scalp. The currents generated are called electrical potentials and together make brain waves. Put electrodes on the scalp to measure the electrical currents and you get an electroencephalogram (EEG). That test shows us the location and coordination of electrical energy produced by brain cells in response to stimulation or during a particular activity. Brain wave patterns are different when awake versus asleep. In fact the EEG has a characteristic signature pattern for each different stage of sleep. That is partly how we can determine sleep stages during a sleep study.

So studying brain waves provides much information about brain function. No, you can't see someone's thoughts. But you can infer what particular part the brain is active during specific activities.

Brain Function

Let's start at the very beginning.

It is a remarkable thing this brain we have. It is hugely more complicated than even the most sophisticated computer that has yet been created. It controls our entire body, which is also incredibly complex. It takes what we see, hear, smell, taste, and feel and makes sense of it. It controls our movements. The brain also regulates breathing, heart rate, body temperature, digestion, and all of the functions that keep us alive. The brain is arranged very specifically for its functions, which has something to do with sleep function as well.

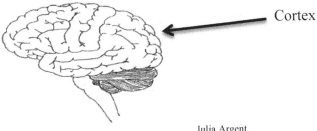 Cortex

Julia Argent

The parts of the brain you usually see in pictures and movies and drawings (like that one up there), is called the CORTEX. It is provides interpretation of the environment and control of how we respond to it. It is here that movements are orchestrated so you don't trip walking down the street. All of the sensory input we get, moment to moment, is recognized and acknowledged here.

217

Managing this information allows us to be able to react to the world, plan our next move, or just sit back and relax. All of our thoughts are generated here as well. Decision-making, new ideas, bad ideas, crazy ideas, calculations, reading and comprehension, planning, complaining…all these things occur at the surface of the brain, the cortex, when you are awake.

Each part of the brain communicates with all of the other parts. The amount of coordination is astounding. Say you hear a bird in the tree above you. The auditory (hearing) cortex senses that sound and coordinates with the frontal cortex for recognition that you have heard a bird. A signal is sent to the motor cortex area to move your head upward to try to see that bird. The eyes, that are controlled deeper in the brain stem, move in coordination with your head upward to find it in the tree. The messages from the eyes come in to the back of the brain where vision is sensed. That image is processed and a message is sent to the front again. Yup, Blue Jay up there.

Imagine the efficiency and power of the brain. A major league hitter has a split second to decide whether to swing when he sees a 90 mph fastball leave a pitcher's hand. Einstein's brain came up with a theory, never before discovered about time and space, by piecing together the evidence in a unique way no one had ever done. The brain is pretty amazing.

So now you are done hitting a hanging curve ball and reconsidering the cosmos. It has been a long day. You don't need to be thinking and seeing and smelling and moving when you are sleeping. You need to turn off most of that stuff off so you can get some Z's. It is the deeper and, as the anatomists eerily say, more primitive parts of the brain that shut all of these higher functions down. How does that occur? Let's take a look.

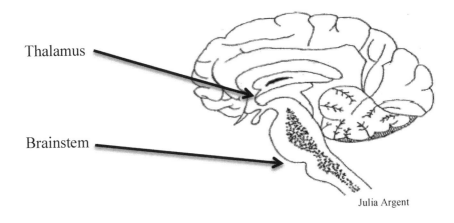

Thalamus

Brainstem

Julia Argent

The brainstem (which includes the midbrain, the pons and reticular formation) and the thalamus (and surrounding structures like the hypothalamus, pituitary, pineal body and mammillary bodies) are extremely important structures. (See illustration of a brain cut in half to reveal these structures, above.) It is in these areas that the non-thinking activities of our bodies are controlled. Our body temperature, heart rate, breathing, and digestion, all of the things that happen without our conscious input, are coordinated here. These are the functions that keep us alive and kicking. No higher thoughts, or artistic expression; just making sure that the machinery is working correctly. Don't get too caught up in the names and locations of these structures. You can see that this is a very complicated part of the body.

Now lets talk sleep, which is also one of those critical functions controlled deep in the brain. What brain chemicals (neurotransmitters) these areas produce, and how these structures interact, is where the sleep action is. Some of these areas are sleep inducing, some are wake promoting, and some play a part in both sides of the sleep equation.

Lets start with the areas that keep us awake and the chemicals that they produce to accomplish that task. Bear with me here. It gets pretty ugly with all of these names and locations. It will make sense soon enough if you are patient.

The awake areas and their neurotransmitters are as follows (see illustration below):

Basal forebrain	Acetyl Choline (ACh)
Tuberomamillary nucleus	Histamine (HA)
Ventral gray areas	Dopamine (DA)
Raphe nuclei	Sertonin (5-HT)
Locus coeruleus	Norepinephrine (NE)
Hypothalamus	Orexin (who didn't get an abbreviation)

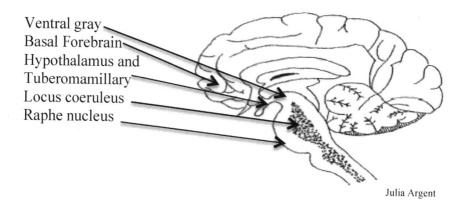

Julia Argent

Again, please don't get bogged down on those names. The point is that these areas, located deep in the brain, connect to the cortex. The message they send through their neurotransmitters is "wake up and stay awake!" Why is this information important? Look at the chemical messengers. You may recognize some of the names. Histamine, dopamine, and epinephrine – all are chemicals that are manipulated for treatment of health problems. When we talk about how medicines and illnesses impact sleep, we can usually point to an effect on one of those chemicals to explain the problem.

Okay, so there are areas that wake us and keep us up. What parts make us go to sleep, you might ask? The sleep promoters, much smaller in number but just as important, are as follows (see illustration below):

Preoptic area

Pineal gland

Gamma aminobutyric
acid (GABA)

Melatonin

Pineal Gland

Preoptic Area

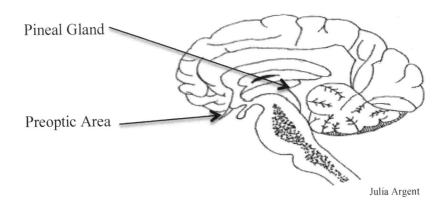

Julia Argent

These chemical messengers go to the wake areas and shut them down. When the "wake up" messages to the cortex are gone, we sleep.

Whether you are awake or asleep has to do with the balance between these areas. During the day we are conscious and those wake promoters predominate. They inhibit, or turn off, the sleep promoters. At night it is the other way around. Those sleep areas turn off the wake areas very quickly and efficiently. It really is lights out before you know it. One minute you are reading or watching the news, conversing and thinking. The next you are asleep. This rapid transition from being awake to asleep, and vice versa, is controlled very cleverly.

The balance between these dueling systems is a really cool story.

The suprachiasmatic nucleus (SCN) is the key. Another big name, but it means something to your understanding of sleep. Let's break it down. "Supra" indicates above. "Chiasmatic " refers to the area where the optic nerves (those that carry visual information from the eyes to the visual brain cortex) cross, or their chiasm. That they cross is less important than the information they carry.

221

Visual input is all about light, or lack thereof. And it is light that helps regulate our sleep/wake cycles. So this nucleus (or group of brain/nerve cells) is positioned perfectly by sitting on top of the nerves where it can pick up light cues about day and night. It is here that our internal clock lives. It is from here that our sleep is turned off and on.

You may have heard the term "circadian rhythm" before. "Circa" means around, and "dian" refers to day. This cadence is the daily rhythm of our lives. It controls temperature changes, hormone levels, bodily functions, and is one of the main drivers of our need to sleep. It has a time period of about, but not exactly, 24 hours. This may seem odd because our lives revolve around that 24 hour day. However, in most animals studied, including humans, the natural circadian time period is just over 24 hours. So we need more than just those cells timing our days and nights. That is where light comes in.

Included in the optic nerve are some special fibers that go from the eye directly to the SCN. These nerves carry information about how light or dark it is in the environment. It is this light information that resets the internal clock every day to sync with our 24 hour world.

Here is where it gets cool. When it begins to get dark outside, the SCN gets busy. It sends a message to the Pineal Gland to produce to melatonin, a sleep hormone that signals the circadian "end of the day." This prepares the brain and body for the upcoming night of sleep. When night finally falls, the internal clock in the SCN delivers a message to the Pre-Optic area, which in turn sends out GABA to quickly turn off those awake-promoting areas of the brain.

After we are asleep Melatonin works similarly to GABA. It helps keep us asleep by blocking those wake promoting pathways. It is a very sensitive system. Exposure to light during the night sharply, and within 5 minutes, decreases Melatonin production **(Prasai)** to disrupt sleep.

In the morning, as light increases, the SCN stops promoting sleep. The balance shifts back to being awake.

But it is not only the circadian rhythm and the Suprachiasmatic Nucleus that controls sleep. There is more – the metabolic sleep drive.

After an entire day of being CEO of your body, your brain gets tired, just like the rest of the body. When you exercise your muscles get tired. Energy stores are used up and you need to rest so that your strength returns. Your brain needs the same thing.

For a long time scientists couldn't figure out what it was that made the brain feel tired, mentally. There was this mysterious "Substance S" that seemed to build up in the brain and induce sleep. It was most powerful in the early part of the night and wore off as the night wore on. We have now identified "Substance S" and it makes a lot of sense. Follow along and it should all become clear.

Glucose sugar is the energy supply of the brain. A chemical called Adenosine is the rechargeable battery of the body. Glucose is the power plant that fuels Adenosine, recharging the battery used to energize brain function. It is a complex chemical reaction that occurs in brain cells, but it goes something like this. Enzymes in the cells break down glucose sugar, releasing its energy. Phosphate molecules take that energy with them as they attach themselves to Adenosine. Once an Adenosine molecule has 3 phosphates attached (adenosine triphosphate – ATP), it is fully charged and ready to fuel the activities of the brain. The ATP goes around providing energy for all of the cell's activities. In other words, ATP is the energy delivery system. Usable energy is released by removing phosphate molecules from the Adenosine. As the brain uses up its energy stores ATP levels decrease and Adenosine levels increase.

There is your mysterious "Substance S," Adenosine. Having lots of Adenosine around means that energy stores are low and the brain needs to rest and recharge. We call this the Metabolic drive to sleep. Metabolism slows, sleep happens. When you go to sleep the brain recharges its batteries by recharging the adenosine back to ATP, and that sleepiness goes away. Pretty slick.

We have two separate and complementary systems that make us feel like we need to sleep. One is brain weariness, really the build up of Adenosine, that signals sleepiness at the beginning of the night. The second is the circadian drive, timing the day/night cycle, keeping us asleep once our batteries have recharged, and using light to reset our clocks to an awake pattern in the morning.

We are not slaves to these rhythms. As thinking beings there are lots of things under our control that influence our sleep. We have a lot to say about when and how much we sleep. We can consciously decide to stay awake despite our body's signals. Emotions, illnesses, pains, medicines, sleep situations, stressors, and distractions all influence our sleep or lack thereof. In fact NOT getting enough sleep is what most of this book is about.

References

Chapter 2: Advice for Smarter Sleep

Campbell, S. Effects of a month-long napping regimen in older individuals. J Am Geriatr Soc. 2011;59(2):224-32.

Milner, C. Benefits of napping in healthy adults: impact of nap length, time of day, age, and experience with napping. Journal of Sleep Research. 2009;18(2):272–281.

Myliymaki, T. Effects of vigorous late-night exercise on sleep quality and cardiac autonomic activity. J. Sleep Res. 2011;20: 146–153.

NSF. www.sleepfoundation.org.

Rahman, S. Diurnal Spectral Sensitivity of the Acute Alerting Effects of Light. Sleep. 2014;37(2):271-281.

Stein, M. Disturbed Sleep and Its Relationship to Alcohol Use. Subst Abus. 2005;26(1):1–13.

Youngstedt, S. From Wake to Sleep. The Effects of Acute Exercise on Sleep: A Quantitative Synthesis. Sleep. 1997; 20(3):203-214.

Chapter 3: Insomnia

Bennett, T. Suvorexant, a Dual Orexin Receptor Antagonist for the Management of Insomnia. P&T®. 2014; 39(4): 264-266.
CBS News. "Sleeping pill use tied to higher death risk. People taking most pills may be more likely than smokers to get some cancers." Posted: Feb 28, 2012 2:38 PM ET.

Krystal, A. Efficacy and Safety of Doxepin 1 mg and 3 mg in a 12-week Sleep Laboratory and Outpatient Trial of Elderly Subjects with Chronic Primary Insomnia. Sleep.2010; 33(11): 1553-1561.

NSF. http://www.sleepfoundation.org/article/sleep-related-problems/sleep-aids-and-insomnia.

Qi, S. Clinical and Familial Characteristics of Ten Chinese Patients with Fatal Family Insomnia. Biomed Environ Sci, 2012; 25(4):471-475.

Ringdahl, E. Treatment of Primary Insomnia. J Am Board Fam Med. 2004;17(3):212-219

Sateia, M. Evaluation Of Chronic Insomnia, An American Academy Of Sleep Medicine Review. SLEEP. 2000;23(2):243-308.

Sun H. Effects of suvorexant, an orexin receptor antagonist, on sleep parameters as measured by polysomnography in healthy men. SLEEP. 2013;36(2):259-267.

Chapter 4: Snoring

Brietzke, S. Injection snoreplasty: Extended follow-up and new objective data. Otolaryngol Head Neck Surg 2003;128:605-15.

Carroll, W. Snoring Management with Nasal Surgery and Upper Airway Radiofrequency Ablation. Otolaryngology–Head and Neck Surgery 146(6):1023-1027.

Doff, M. Oral appliance versus continuous positive airway pressure in Obstructive Sleep Apnea Syndrome: a 2-year follow-up. SLEEP 2013:36(9):1289-1296.

Hoffstein, V. Review of oral appliances for treatment of sleep-disordered breathing. Sleep Breath (2007) 11:1–22.

Hsueh-Y, L. Improvement in Quality of Life After Nasal Surgery Alone for Patients With Obstructive Sleep Apnea and Nasal Obstruction. Arch Otolaryngol Head Neck Surg. 2008;134(4):429-433.

Lazard, D. The Tongue-Retaining Device: Efficacy and Side Effects in Obstructive Sleep Apnea Syndrome. J Clin Sleep Med 2009;5(5):431-438.

Macdonald, A. Evaluation of Potential Predictors of Outcome of Laser-Assisted Uvulopalatoplasty for Snoring. Otolaryngology–Head and Neck Surgery. 2006;134:197-203.

Medical Advisory Secretariat. Oral appliances for obstructive sleep apnea: an evidence-based analysis.

Ontario Health Technology Assessment Series 2009;9(5):31.

Rappai, M. The Nose and Sleep-Disordered Breathing.* What We Know and What We Do Not Know. CHEST 2003;124:2309–2323.

Rosenthal, L. A Multicenter, Prospective Study of a Novel Nasal EPAP Device in the Treatment of Obstructive Sleep Apnea: Efficacy and 30-Day Adherence. J Clin Sleep Med;5(6):532-537.

Stale, N. Palatal implants for the treatment of snoring: Long-term resultsOtolaryngology–Head and Neck Surgery. 2006;134(4):558-564.

Stapleton, A. The Impact of Nasal Surgery on Sleep Quality: A Prospective Outcomes Study. Otolaryngology–Head and Neck Surgery. 2014;151(5):868–873.

227

Wong, L. Decrease of resistance to air flow with nasal strips as measured with the airflow perturbation device. *BioMedical Engineering OnLine* 2004;3:38.

Chapter 5: Obstructive Sleep Apnea

Aurora, R. Practice Parameters for the Surgical Modifications of the Upper Airway for Obstructive Sleep Apnea in Adults. Sleep. 2010;33(10):1408–1413.

Ayappa, I. Validation of a Self-Applied Unattended Monitor for Sleep Disordered Breathing. J Clin Sleep Med. 2008; 4(1): 26–37.

Camacho, M., et al. "The Effect of Nasal Surgery on Continuous Positive Airway Pressure Device Use and Therapeutic Treatment Pressures: A Systematic Review and Meta-Analysis." SLEEP 2015;38(2):279–286.

Caples, SM, et al. "Surgical Modifications of the Upper Airway for Obstructive Sleep Apnea in Adults: A Systematic Review and Meta-Analysis." SLEEP 2010;33(10):1396-1407.

Dehidia, R. "Upper Airway Stimulation for Obstructive Sleep Apnea: Past, Present, and Future." SLEEP 2015;38(6): 899-906. Doff, M. Oral appliance versus continuous positive airway pressure in Obstructive Sleep Apnea: a 2-year follow-up. SLEEP 2013;36(9):1289-1296.

Friedman, M. Transoral robotic glossectomy for the treatment of Obstructive Sleep Apnea-Hypopnea Syndrome. Otolaryngology– Head and Neck Surgery. 2012;146(5):854–862.

Hoffstein, V. Review of oral appliances for treatment of sleep-disordered breathing. Sleep Breath 2007;11:1-22.

Howard, ME, et al. Sleepiness, Sleep-disordered Breathing, and Accident Risk Factors in Commercial Vehicle Drivers. Am J Respir Crit Care Med. 2004;170:1014–1021.

Inoue Y. Efficacy and safety of adjunctive modafinil treatment on residual excessive daytime sleepiness among nasal continuous positive airway pressure-treated Japanese patients with obstructive sleep apnea syndrome: a double-blind placebo-controlled study. J Clin Sleep Med 2013;9(8):751-757.

Inspire. www.inspiresleep.com

Kushida, CA. Clinical guidelines for the manual titration of positive airway pressure in patients with obstructive sleep apnea. J Clin Sleep Med. 2008;15;4(2):157-71.

Li, K.K.Long-term Results of Maxillomandibular Advancement Surgery. Sleep and Breathing 2000;4(3):137-140.

Marin, J.M. Association Between Treated and Untreated Obstructive Sleep Apnea and Risk of Hypertension JAMA. 2012;307(20);2169-2176.

Naraghi, M. Quality of life comparison in common rhinologic surgeries. Allergy Rhinol. 2010; 3:e1–e7.
Plzak, J. Combined bipolar radiofrequency surgery of the tongue base and uvulopalatopharyngoplasty for obstructive sleep apnea. Arch Med Sci 2013;9(6):1097–1101.

Pollan, M. The Omnivore's Dilemma. Penguin Press, 2006.
Steward, D. Safety and Effectiveness of Upper Airway Stimulation via the Hypoglossal Nerve for Obstructive Sleep Apnea. Otolaryngology–Head and Neck Surgery. 2013;149(2S):13.

Punjabi, N. The Epidemiology of Adult Obstructive Sleep Apnea. Proc Am Thorac Soc. 2008;5:136–143.

Strollo, P. Upper-Airway Stimulation for Obstructive Sleep Apnea. N Engl J Med 2014; 370:139-149

Veasey, S. Medical therapy for Obstructive Sleep Apnea: A review by the medical therapy for Obstructive Sleep Apnea Task Force of the Standards of Practice Committee of the American Academy of Sleep Apnea. SLEEP 2006;29(8):1036-1044.

Yin, SK. Genioglossus advancement and hyoid suspension plus uvulopalatopharyngoplasty for severe OSAHS. Otolaryngology - Head and Neck Surgery 2007;136:626-631.

Chapter 6: Central Sleep Apnea

Brown, S. A Retrospective Case Series of Adaptive Servoventilation for Complex Sleep Apnea. J Clin Sleep Med. 2011;7(2):187-195.

Malhotra, A. What Is Central Sleep Apnea? Respir Care 2010;55(9):1168 –1176.

Patwari P. Congenital central hypoventilation syndrome and the PHOX2B gene: a model of respiratory and autonomic dysregulation. Respir Physiol Neurobiol. 2010;173(3):322-35.

Chapter 7: Circadian Rhythm Disorders

Barion, A. A Clinical Approach to Circadian Rhythm Sleep Disorders. Sleep Med. 2007;8(6):566–577.
Beaumont, M. Caffeine or melatonin effects on sleep and sleepiness after rapid eastward transmeridian travel. *J Appl Physiol*. 2004;96:50–58.

Cattarall, J. ABC of sleep disorders. Nocturnal asthma. BMJ. 1993;306(6886):1189–1192.

Chesson A. Practice parameters for the use of light therapy in the treatment of sleep disorders. Standards of Practice Committee. American Academy of Sleep Medicine Sleep 1999;22(5):641–60.

Dodson, E. Therapeutics for Circadian Rhythm Sleep Disorders. Sleep Med Clin. 2010;5(4):701–715.

Drake, C. Sleep. Shift work sleep disorder: prevalence and consequences beyond that of symptomatic day workers. 2004;27(8):1453-62.

Eastman, C. Advancing Circadian Rhythms Before Eastward Flight: A Strategy to Prevent or Reduce Jet Lag. Sleep. 2005; 28(1): 33–44.

Huang, W. Circadian Rhythms, Sleep, and Metabolism. The Journal of Clinical Investigation. June 2011;121(6):2133-2141.

van Geijlswijk I. The use of exogenous melatonin in delayed sleep phase disorder: a meta-analysis. SLEEP 2010;33(12):1605-1614.

Prasai, M. An Endocrinologist Guide to the Clock. J Clin Endocrinol Metab. 20011;96: 913–922.

Routledge, F.Night-time blood pressure patterns and target organ damage: A review. Can J Cardiol. 2007; 23(2):132–138.

Sack R. Circadian rhythm sleep disorders: Part I, basic principles, shift work and jet lag disorders. SLEEP 2007;30(11):1460-1483.

Auger, R. Sleep Related Eating Disorders. Psychiatry, Psychiatry (Edgmont) 2006;3(11):64–70).

Horn, M. Boston College Law Review, Volume 46Issue 1 Number 1,12-1-2004. A Rude Awakening: What to Do with the Sleepwalking Defense?

Guardian Newspaper. http://www.guardian.co.uk/uk/2009/nov/20/brian-thomas-dream-strangler-tragedy.

Guilleminault, C. Atypical Sexual Behavior During Sleep. Psychosomatic Medicine. 2002;64:328–336.

Ibrahim, I. Somnambulistic sexual behaviour (sexsomnia). Journal of Clinical Forensic Medicine. Volume 13, Issue 4, Pages 219-224, May 2006.

IMBD. http://www.imdb.com/title/tt0120147/plotsummary.

NIH. http://www.ninds.nih.gov/disorders/kleine_levin/kleine _levin.htm

Ohahon, MM. Violent Behavior During Sleep: Prevalence, Comorbidity, and Consequences. Sleep Med. 2010;11(9): 941-946.

Pressman, MR. Disorders of Arousal from Sleep and Violent Behavior: the Role of Physical Contact and Proximity. Sleep. 2007. 30(8):1039-1047.

Schenck CH. Additional Categories of Sleep-Related Eating Disorders and the Current Status of Treatment. Sleep. 1993; 16(5):467-466.

Schenck, CH, et al. Sleep and Sex: What Can Go Wrong? A Review of the Literature on Sleep Related Disorders and Abnormal Sexual Behaviors and Experiences. SLEEP, 2007; 30(6):683-702.

Chapter 9: Movements That Wake You Up: (A.K.A Dancin' the Watusi - Or Not)

Aurora, RN. The treatment of restless legs syndrome and periodic limb movement disorder in adults—an update for 2012: practice parameters with an evidence-based systematic review and meta-analyses. *SLEEP* 2012;35(8):1039-1062.

Brindani, F. Restless legs syndrome: differential diagnosis and management with pramipexole. Clin Interv Aging. 2009;4:305–313.

Buchfuhrer, M. Strategies for the Treatment of Restless Legs Syndrome. Neurotherapeutics. 2012;9:776–790

Fukada, K. High Prevalence Of Isolated Sleep Paralysis: Kanashibari Phenomenon In Japan. Sleep, 10(3):279-286.

Sharpless, B. Lifetime Prevalence Rates of Sleep Paralysis: A Systematic Review. Sleep Med Rev. 2011;15(5):311–315.

Silber MH; Girish M; Izurieta R. Pramipexole in the management of restless legs syndrome: an extended study. SLEEP 2003;26(7):819-21.

Chapter 10: The Hallucination Parasomnias (A.K.A.- "What the ...?)

Cheyne, J. Relations among hypnagogic and hypnopompic experiences associated with sleep paralysis. *J. Sleep Res.*1999; 8:313–317.

Kompanje E. 'The devil lay upon her and held her down'. Hypnagogic hallucinations and sleep paralysis described by the Dutch physician Isbrand van Diemerbroeck (1609-1674) in 1664. J Sleep Res. 2008;17(4):464-7.

Sachs, C. The Exploding Head Syndrome: Polysomnographic Recordings and Therapeutic Suggestions. SLEEP. 1991;14(3):263-266.

Chapter 11: REM Associated Parasomnias

Aurora RN; Zak RS; Auerbach SH; Casey KR. Best practice guide for the treatment of nightmare disorder in adults. J Clin Sleep Med. 2010;6(4):389-401.

Fukuda, K. High Prevalence Of Isolated Sleep Paralysis: Kanashibari Phenomenon In Japan. Sleep 10(3):279-286.

Kierlin, L. Parasomnias and antidepressant therapy: a review of the literature. Frontiers in Psychiatry. 2011;(2)1:1-8.

Trotti. REM Behavior Disorder in Older IndividualsDrugs Aging. 2010;27(6):457–470.

Chapter 12: Enuresis

Kramer, N. Enuresis and Obstructive Sleep Apnea in Adults. Chest 1998;114:634-637.

NAFC. National Association for Continence. www.nafc.org/bladder-bowel-health/bedwetting-2/adult-bedwetting.

Whiteside, C. Persistent Primary Enuresis: A urodynamic Assessment. BMJ 1975;1:364-367.

234

Chapter 13: Narcolepsy and the Hypersomnias (Dig that funky sound)

Black, J. The Nightly Use of Sodium Oxybate Is Associated with a Reduction in Nocturnal Sleep Disruption: A Double-Blind, Placebo-Controlled Study in Patients with Narcolepsy. J Clin Sleep Med. 2010;6(6):596-602.

Mignot, E. A Practical Guide to the Therapy of Narcolepsy and Hypersomnia Syndromes. Neurotherapeutics (2012);9:739–752.

NINDS. National Institute of Neurologic Disorders and Stroke. http://www.ninds.nih.gov/disorders/kleine_levin/kleine_levin.ht m

Ramgurg, S. Kleine-Levin Syndrome: Etiology, diagnosis, and treatment. Ann Indian Acad Neurol. 2010;13(4):241-246.

Wise, M. Treatment of Narcolepsy and other Hypersomnias of Central Origin. SLEEP 2007;30(12):1712-1727.

Chapter 14: Medical Problems and Sleep

Agusti, A. Night-time symptoms: a forgotten dimension of COPD. Eur Respir Rev. 2011;20(12):1183-194.

Al-Jahdali, H. Insomnia in chronic renal patients on dialysis in Saudi Arabia. Journal of Circadian Rhythms. 2010;8(7):1-7.

Anacoli-Israel, S. The Effect of Nocturia on Sleep. Sleep Med Rev. 2011;15(2): 91–97.

Arnold, L. Improving the Recognition and Diagnosis of Fibromyalgia. Mayo Clin Proc. 2011;86(5):457-464.

Arnulf. Sleep Disorders and Diaphragmatic Function in Patients with Amyotrophic Lateral Sclerosis. Am J Respir Crit Care Med. 2000;161:849–856.

Bennett, R. An internet survey of 2,596 people with fibromyalgia. BMC Musculoskeletal Disorders. 2007;8:27:1-11.

Beyenburg, S. Anxiety in patients with epilepsy: Systematic review and suggestions for clinical management. Epilepsy & Behavior ;7(2005):161–171.

Boomershine. Pregabalin for the Management of Fibromyalgia Syndrome. J Pain Res. 2010;22;3:81-88.

Braley, T. Fatigue in Multiple Sclerosis: Mechanisms, Evaluation, and Treatment. Sleep. 2010;33(8):1061-1067.

Brindini, F. Restless legs syndrome: differential diagnosis and management with pramipexole. Clinical Interventions In Aging. 2009;4:305-313.

Campos, MPO. Cancer-related fatigue: a practical review. Annals of Oncology. 2001;22:1273–1279.

Cattaral, J. ABC of sleep disorders. Nocturnal Asthma. BMJ. 1993;306(6886):1189–1192.

Ceko, M. Neurobiology Underlying Fibromyalgia Symptoms. Pain Res Treat. 2012;2012:585419.

Chelimsky G. Co-morbidities of Interstitial Cystitis. Front. Neurosci. 2012;(6)114:1-6.

de Haas S; Exploratory polysomnographic evaluation of pregabalin on sleep disturbance in patients with epilepsy. J Clin Sleep Med. 2007;3(5):473-478.

Deschenes. Current Treatments for Sleep Disturbances in Individuals With Dementia. Curr Psychiatry Rep. 2009;11(1):20–26.

De Simone, R. Hypnic headache: an update. Neurol Sci. 2006; 27:S144–S148.

Ezzie, M. Sleep and Obstructive Lung Diseases. Sleep Med Clin. 2008;3(4):505–515.

French, LM. Interstitial Cystitis/Painful Bladder Syndrome. Am Fam Physician. 2011;83(10):1175-1181.

Ganguly G. "Alarm clock" headaches. J Clin Sleep Med 2011;7(6):681-682.

Hauser, W. Fibromyalgia Syndrome. Dtsch Arztebl Int. 2009;106(23):383–391.

Hussein. Adjuvant use of melatonin for treatment of fibromyalgia. J Pineal Res. 2011;50(3):267-71.

Junqueira , P. Women living With HIV/AIDS, Sleep impairment, anxiety and depression symptoms. Neuropsiquiatr 2008;66(4):817-820.

Kalish, R. Evaluation of Study Patients with Lyme Disease, 10–20-Year Follow-up. J. Inf. Dis. 2001;183:453-460.
Krishnan, V., et al. Sleep Quality and Health-Related Quality of Life in Idiopathic Pulmonary Fibrosis. CHEST 2008;134:693–698.

Kwekkeboom,, KL. Mind-Body Treatments for the Pain-Fatigue-Sleep Disturbance. Symptom Cluster in Persons with Cancer. J Pain Symptom Manage. 2010 ; 39(1):126–138.

Lavery C. Nonuniform nighttime distribution of acute cardiac events: A possible effect of sleep states. Circulation. 1997;5:3321–3327.

Lee K. Types of sleep problems in adults living with HIV/AIDS. J Clin Sleep Med. 2012;8(1):67-75.

Lee, K. Symptom Experience in HIV-Infected Adults: A Function of Demographic and Clinical Characteristics. J Pain Symptom Manage. 2009; 38(6):882–893.

Logigian, E. Chronic Neurologic Manifestations of Lyme Disease. NEJM. 1990;323:1438-44.

Malow, B. Approach to daytime sleepiness. SLEEP. 1995;18(9):783-786.

Martin, J. Sleep Disturbances in Long-term Care. Clin Geriatr Med. 2008;24(1):39–vi.

Menza, M. Sleep Disturbances in Parkinson's Disease. Mov Disord. 2010;25(Suppl 1):S117–S122.

Mukerji V. Dyspnea, Orthopnea, and Paroxysmal Nocturnal Dyspnea. In: Walker, HK, Hall WD, Hurst JW, editors. Clinical Methods: The History, Physical, and Laboratory Examinations. 3rd edition. Boston: Butterworths; 1990. Chapter 11. Available from: http://www.ncbi.nlm.nih.gov/books/NBK213/.

Newsom-Davis. The effect of non-invasive positive pressure ventilation (NIPPV) on cognitive function in amyotrophic lateral sclerosis (ALS): a prospective study. J Neurol Neurosurg Psychiatry. 2001;71:482–487.

Ondo. Exploring the Relationship Between Parkinson's disease and Restless Legs Syndrome. Arch Neurol 2002;59:421-424.

Parish, J. Sleep-Related Problems in Common Medical Conditions. CHEST. 2009;135;563-572.

Pellegrino, R. CPAP as a novel treatment for bronchial asthma? J Appl Physiol. 2011;111(2):343-344.

Penzel, T. Dynamics of Heart Rate and Sleep Stages in Normals and Patients with Sleep Apnea. Neuropsychopharmacology (2003)28:S48–S53.

Rasche, K. Sleep and Breathing in Idiopathic Pulmonary Fibrosis. J Phys Pharm. 2009;60(Suppl. 5):13-14.

Routledge, F. Night-time blood pressure patterns and target organ damage: A review. Can J Cardiol. 2007; 23(2): 132–138.

Schuiling, WJ. Disorders of Sleep and Wake in Patients After Subarachnoid Hemorrhage. Stroke. 2005;36:578-582.

Teodorescu, M. Association of Obstructive Sleep Apnea Risk With Asthma Control in Adults. Chest. 2010;138(3): 543–550.

Teroni, L. Importance of retardation and fatigue/interest domains for the diagnosis of major depressive episode after stroke: a four months prospective study Rev Bras Psiquiatr. 2009;31(3):202-7.

Trotti. REM Sleep Behaviour Disorder in Older Individuals: Epidemiology, Pathophysiology, and Management. Drugs Aging. 2010;27(6):457–470.

Verrier, R. Impact of Sleep on Arrhythmogenesis. Circ Arrhythm Electrophysiol. 2009;2(4):450–459.

Vock, J. Evolution of sleep and sleep EEG after hemispheric stroke. J. Sleep Res. 2002;11:331–338.

Chapter 15: Psychiatric Problems and Sleep

Abad, V. Sleep and Psychiatry. Diloges Clin Neurosci. 2005;7:291-303.

Abe, Y. Early Sleep psychiatric Intervention for Acute Insomnia: Implications from a Case of obsessive-Compulsive disorder. J Clin Sleep Med 2012;8(2):191-193.

Agarwal, R. The quality of life of adults with Attention Deficit Disorder: a systematic review. Innov Clin Neurosci. 2012;9(5-6):10-21.

Austin, D. Managing panic disorder in general practice. Australian Family Physician. 2005;34(7):563-71.

Dørheim, S. Sleep and Depression in Postpartum Women: A Population-Based Study. SLEEP 2009;32(7):847-855.

Franzen, PL. Sleep disturbances and depression: risk relationships for subsequent depression and therapeutic implications. Dialogues Clin Neurosci. 2008;10:473-481.

Harvey, AG. Sleep Disturbance as Transdiagnostic: Consideration of Neurobiological Mechanisms. Clin Psychol Rev. 2011;31(2):225–235.

Hofstetter, JR. Quality of sleep in patients with schizophrenia is associated with quality of life and coping. BMC Psychiatry 2005;5:13.

Kane, JM Unanswered Question in Schizophrenia Clinical Trials. Schizophrenia Bulletin 2008;34(2):302-309.

Kupfer, DJ. Major depressive disorder: new clinical, neurobiological, and treatment perspectives. Lancet. 2012;379(9820):1045-1055.

Lamont, EW. The role of circadian clock genes in mental disorders. Dialogues Clin Neurosci. 2007;9:333-342.

Lamont EW. Circadian Rhythms and Clock Genes in Psychotic Disorders. Isr J Psychiatriy Rela Sci. 2010;47(1):27-35.

Leboyer, M. Bipolar disorder: new perspectives in health care and prevention. J Clin Psychiatry. 2010;71(12):1689–1695.

Lohoff, FW. Overview of the Genetics of Major Depressive Disorder. Cur. Psychiatry Rep. 2010;12(6):539-546.

Meijer, WM. Current issues around the pharmacotherapy of ADD/ADHD in children and adults. Pharm World Sci. 31(5): 509-516.

Meltzer-Brody, S. New insights into pernatal depression: pathogenesis and treatment during pregnancy and postpartum. Dialogues Clin Neurosci. 2011;13:89-100.

Posmontier, B. Sleep Quality in Women with and without Postpartum Depression. Obstet Gynecol Neonatal Nurs, 2008; 36(6):722-737.

Salvadore , G. The Neurobiology of the Switch Process in Bipolar Disorder: a Review. J Clin Psychiatry. 2010;71(11):1488–1501.

Sharpless, B. Lifetime Prevalence Rates of Sleep Paralysis: A Systematic Review. Sleep Med Rev. 2011;15(5):311–315.

Sobanski E. Sleep in adults with attention deficit hyperactivity disorder (ADHD) before and during treatment with methylphenidate: a controlled polysomnographic study. SLEEP 2007;31(3):375-381.

Staner, L. Sleep and anxiety disorders. Dialogues Clin Neurosci. 2003;5(3):249–258.

van Liempt , S. Sleep disturbances and PTSD: a perpetual circle? European Journal of Psychotraumatology. 2012;3:19142.

Chen, W. Postmenopausal Hormone Therapy and Breast Cancer Risk: Current Status and Unanswered Questions. Endocrinol Metab Clin North Am. 2011;40(3):509–518.

Edwards, B. Aging and Sleep: Physiology and Pathophysiology. Semin Respir Crit Care Med. 2010;31(5):618-633.

Girard, T. Delirium in the intensive care unit. Crit Care. 2008; 12(Suppl 3):S3.

Kravitz, H. Sleep During the Perimenopause: A SWAN Story. Obstet Gynecol Clin North Am. 2011;38(3):567–586.

Martin, J. Sleep Disturbances in Long-term Care. Clin Geriatr Med. 2008;24(1):39-vi.

Neikrug, A. Sleep Disorders in the Older Adult – A Mini-Review. Gerontology. 2010;56(2):181–189.

Punjabi, N. The Epidemiology of Adult Obstructive Sleep Apnea. Proc Am Thorac Soc. 2008;5(2):136–143.

Sanders, R. Contribution of sedative-hypnotic agents to delirium via modulation of the sleep pathway. Can J Anaesth. 2011;58(2):149-156.

Utian, W. Psychosocial and socioeconomic burden of vasomotor symptoms in menopause: A comprehensive review. Health and Quality of Life Outcomes 2005, 3:47.

Weinhaus, G. Bench-to-bedside review: Delerium in ICU patients – importance of sleep deprivation. Crit Care. 2009;13(6):234.

Wolkove, N. Sleep and aging: Sleep disorders commonly found in older people. CMAJ. 2007;176(9):1299–1304.

Chapter 17: Medications and Sleep

Adam, K. The hypnotic effects of an antihistamine: promethazine. Br J Clin Pharmacol. 1986;22(6):715–717.

Arendt, J. Sleep Following Alcohol Intoxication in Healthy, Young Adults: Effects of Sex and Family History of Alcoholism. Alcohol Clin Exp Res. 2011;35(5):870–878.

Arria, A. Nonmedical Use of Prescription Stimulants Among Students. Pediatr Ann. 2006;35(8):565–571.

Aurora RN, et al. Best practice guide for the treatment of nightmare disorder in adults. J Clin Sleep Med. 2010;6(4):389-401.

Dionysus. http://www.theoi.com/Olympios/DionysosGod.html.

Bonnet. Stimulants and Sleep Loss. SLEEP. 2005;28(9);1163-1187.

Boomershine. Pregabalin for the Management of Fibromyalgia Syndrome. J Pain Res. 2010;22(3):81-8.

Brower, K. Persistent insomnia, abstinence, and moderate drinking in alcohol-dependent individuals. Am J Addict. 2011;20(5): 435–440.

Bostwick, J. A Generalist's Guide to Treating Patients With Depression With an Emphasis on Using Side Effects to Tailor Antidepressant Therapy. Mayo Clin Proc. 2010;85(6):538-550.

Chong, Y. Prescription sleep aid use among adults: United States, 2005–2010. NCHS data brief, no 127. Hyattsville, MD: National Center for Health Statistics. 2013.

Dimsdale, J. The Effect of Opioids on Sleep Architecture. J Clin Sleep Med. 2007;3(1):33-36.

Farney, R. Sleep-Disordered Breathing Associated With Long-term Opioid Therapy. CHEST. 2003;123:632–639.

Fernandez-Mendoza, J. Clinical and Polysomnographic Predictors of the Natural History of Poor Sleep. SLEEP. 2012;35(5):689-697.

Ferreira, J. Effect of ropinirole on sleep onset: A randomized, placebo controlled study in healthy volunteers. Neurology 2002;58:460–462.

IMS Health, National Prescription Audit, Dec 2010.

Informer. http://www.caffeineinformer.com/the-caffeine-database

Jasinski, D. An evaluation of the abuse potential of modafinil using methylphenidate as a reference. J Psychopharm. 2000;14(1):53–60.

Kelly, K. Toward achieving optimal response: understanding and managing antidepressant side effects. Dialogues Clin Neurosci. 2008;10:409-418.

Lakhan, S. Prescription stimulants in individuals with and without attention deficit hyperactivity disorder: misuse, cognitive impact, and adverse effects. Brain and Behavior. 2012; 2(5): 661–677.

Lai, L. Prevalence and factors associated with off-label antidepressant prescriptions for insomnia. Drug, Healthcare and Patient Safety. 2011:3 27–36.

Muench, J. Adverse Effects of Antipsychotic Medications. Am Fam Physician. 2010;81(5):617-622.

Neubauer, D. A review of ramelteon in the treatment of sleep disorders. Neuropsychiatric Disease and Treatment. 2008:4(1) 69–79.

Neubauer, D. Medication Effects on Sleep. ACCP Sleep Medicine Review Course, 2008. Pp. 117-121. http://books.google.com/books?id=kValrmJrl2kC&lpg=PA117& ots=n_yxk_ZeAU&dq=antiarrhythmics%20and%20sleep%20dis ruption&lr&pg=PA118#v=onepage&q=antiarrhythmics%20and %20sleep%20disruption&f=true.

Pagel, J. Medications for the Treatment of Sleep Disorders: An Overview. Prim Care Companion J Clin Psych. 2001;3(3):118-125.

Proctor, A. Clinical Pharmacology in Sleep Medicine. International Scholarly Research Network ISRN Pharmacology Volume 2012 (2012), Article ID 914168

Roehrs, T. Drug-related Sleep Stage Changes: Functional Significance and Clinical Relevance. Sleep Med Clin. 2010;5(4): 559-570.

Roth, T. Evaluation of the Safety of Modafinil for Treatment of Excessive Sleepiness. J Clin Sleep Med. 2007;3(6):595-602.

Schwartz, JRL. Modafinil in the treatment of excessive sleepiness. Drug Design, Development and Therapy. 2008;2:71–85.
Schweitzer, P. Drugs that Disturb Sleep and Wakefulness, p. 509; in Principles and Practice of Sleep Medicine. ed. Kryger, M.

Seifert, S. Health Effects of Energy Drinks on Children, Adolescents, and Young Adults. Pediatrics. 2011;127:511–528.

Sonka, K. Diagnosis and Management of Central Hypersomnias. Ther Adv Neurol Disord. 2012;5(5):297–305.

245

Stradling, J. Recreational drugs and sleep. BMJ. 1993;306:573-575.

Sun H. Effects of suvorexant, an orexin receptor antagonist, on sleep parameters as measured by polysomnography in healthy men. SLEEP. 2013;36(2):259-267.

Utah. http://www.math.utah.edu/~yplee/fun/caffeine.html

Welsh, C. Medications that can Cause Insomnia. Sleep: A Comprehensive Handbook. Ed. Lee-Chiong, T. 2006, John Wiley and Sons, pp. 103-109.
http://books.google.com/books?hl=en&lr=&id=aNhAk4knmukC
&oi=fnd&pg=PA103&dq=which+asthma+medications+disrupt+
sleep%3F&ots=fRYbTnXbkN&sig=obeXIKwsVAKf3w1nJjLcp
_WyZ3s#v=onepage&q=which%20asthma%20medications%20
disrupt%20sleep%3F&f=false.

Wilens, T. An update on the pharmacotherapy of attention-deficit/hyperactivity disorder in adults. Expert Rev Neurother. 2011;11(10):1443–1465.

Zhang, L. Cigarette Smoking and Nocturnal Sleep Architecture. Am J Epidemiol. 2006;164:529–537.

Chapter 18: Complementary and Alternative Medicines (CAM) and Treatments

Allen JA, et al. Post-epidemic eosinophilia myalgia sundrome associated with L-Tryptophan. Arthritis Rheum. 2011;63(11): 10.1002/art.30514.

Bertisch, S. Use of relaxation techniques and complementary and alternative medicine by adults with insomnia symptoms: results from a national survey. BMC Complementary and Alternative Medicine. 2012;12(Suppl 1):P294.

Cao, H., et al. The Journal of Alternative and Complementary Medicine. 2009;15(11);1171–1186.

Carotenuto, M. Acupressure therapy for insomnia in adolescents: a polysomnographic study. Neuropsychiatric Disease and Treatment. 2013;9:157–162.

Cohen, L. Psychological Adjustment and Sleep Quality in a Randomized Trial of the Effects of a Tibetan Yoga Intervention in Patients with Lymphoma. Cancer 2004;100:2253-60.

George, C. The Effect of L-Tryptophan on Daytime Sleep Latency in Normals: Correlation with Blood Levels. 1989; 12(4):345-353.

Irwin, M. Improving Sleep Quality in Older Adults with Moderate Sleep Complaints: A Randomized Controlled Trial of Tai Chi Chih. *SLEEP*. 2008;31(7):1001-1008.

Kozasa, E. Mind-body interventions for the treatment of insomnia: a review. Rev Bras Psiquiatr. 2010;32(4):437-43.

Mason, L. Electrophysiological Correlates of Higher States of Consciousness During Sleep in Long-Term Practitioners of the Transcendental Meditation Program. *Sleep.* 1997;20(2):102-110.

NIH1. http://nccam.nih.gov/health/sleep/ataglance.htm?nav=gsa

NIH2. http://nccam.nih.gov/health/taichi/introduction.htm.

Ringdahl, E. Treatment of Primary Insomnia. J Am Board Fam Med. 2004;17(3):212-219.

Robinson, N. The evidence for Shiatsu: a systematic review of Shiatsu and acupressure. BMC Complementary and Alternative Medicine .2011;11:88.

Tagaki, H. Enhanced Collagen Synthesis and Transcription by

Peak E, a Contaminant of L-Tryptophan Preparations Associated with the Eosinophilia Myalgia Syndrome. Epidemic J. Clin. Invest. 1995;96:2120-2125.

Taibi, D. A randomized clinical trial of Valerian fails to improve self-report, polysomnographic, and actigraphic sleep in older women with insomnia. Sleep Med. 2009;10(3):319–328.

Taibi, D. A Pilot Study of Gentle Yoga for Sleep Disturbance in Women with Osteoarthritis. Sleep Med. 2011;12(5):512–517.

Yeung, W. Electroacupuncture for Primary Insomnia: A Randomized Controlled Trial. *SLEEP* 2009;32(8):1039-1047.

Zick, S. Preliminary examination of the efficacy and safety of a standardized chamomile extract for chronic primary insomnia: A randomized placebo-controlled pilot study. MC Complementary and Alternative Medicine. 2011;11:78.

Chapter 19: Crazy Quackery and Sleep

Puhan, M. Didgeridoo playing as alternative treatment for obstructive sleep apnoea syndrome: randomised controlled trial. BMJ 2006;332:266.

Chapter 20: The Science of Sleep 101

Prasai, M. An Endocrinologist's Guide to the Clock. J Clin Endocrinol Metab 96: 913–922, 201

Index

A

AASM, 62
Abilify®, 188
acid reflux, 12, 151, 152, 159, 160
Aciphex®, 160
acupressure, 204
acupuncture, 204
Acute Insomnia, 31
acute pain, 149
Adaptive Servoventilation, 101, 102, 230
ADD, 147, 174, 190, 241
Adderall®, 145, 147, 175
adenoid, 82
adenoidectomy, 83
adenosine, 223
adenosine triphosphate, 223
ADHD, 174, 190, 241
Adjustment (Acute) Insomnia, 26
adrenalin, 59, 134, 155, 173, 198
Advair®, 198
Advanced Sleep Phase Syndrome, 109, 169
AHI, 66, 71, 91
airbeds, 9
Alarm Clock Headaches, 163
albuterol, 198, 199
alcohol, 13, 14, 15, 18, 19, 29, 48, 57, 113, 114, 122, 126, 141, 160, 185, 211, 225, 243
Allerga®, 199
allergies, 38, 39, 43, 82
ALS, 162, 163, 238
Alzheimer's, 161, 195
Ambien CR®, 33, 195
Ambien®, 32, 62, 113, 114, 151, 164, 195, 196
American Academy of Sleep Medicine, 62
American Board of Sleep Medicine, vi
aminophylline, 198
amitriptyline, 134, 187, 195
amphetamine- dextroamphetamine), 145
amphetamines, 116, 145
Amyotrophic Lateral Sclerosis, 162, 236
Anafranil®, 132, 187
Anesthesiologist, vii
antidepressants, 149, 171, 186, 187
antiepileptics, 187
antihistamines, 199
antipsychotics, 188
Anxiety, 19, 149, 168, 171, 172, 186, 192, 213, 236
apnea, 19, 39, 40, 41, 51, 52, 53, 55, 58, 59, 60, 64, 65, 66, 67, 68, 69, 70, 71, 72, 73, 74, 76, 77, 78, 80, 81, 83, 84, 85, 86, 87, 88, 89, 91, 92, 93, 94, 96, 97, 101, 102, 103, 127, 138, 152, 161, 164, 165, 166, 169, 180, 186, 192, 193, 208, 209, 210, 211, 212, 229, 230, 239
Apnea Hypopnea Index, 66
app, 24
aripiprazole, 188
armodafinil, 97, 117, 145, 147, 166, 192
Arnold Chiari Malformation, 99
ASPS, 109, 169
assisted living facility, 180
Astepro®, 39
asthma, 106, 151, 152, 198, 200, 230, 236, 238, 239, 246
Astramorph®, 193
ASV, 102
ATP, 223
Attention Deficit Disorder, 145, 174, 240
Attention Deficit Hyperactivity Disorder, 174
auto-titration, 72, 95, 96
aveo TSD®., 41
Axid®, 160
azleastine, 39

B

bedwetting, 118, 137
Belsomra®, 33, 195, 196
Ben and Jerry's®, 13
Benadryl®, 195, 199
Betapace®, 197
Bi-level PAP, 74
Bipolar Disease, 176, 177
bladder, 157
blood pressure, 28, 58, 59, 61, 69, 71, 78, 106, 133, 134, 154, 211, 231, 239
Blue Plate Special, 109
BMI, 53, 54
body mass index, 53
brain, 2, 3, 4, 5, 11, 33, 52, 59, 63, 97, 99, 100, 102, 105, 107, 108, 116, 123, 127, 128, 129, 133, 134, 135, 145, 147, 159, 161, 163, 164, 165, 166, 168, 169, 173, 184, 186, 187, 188, 191, 195, 196, 197, 198, 199, 206, 213, 216, 217, 218, 219, 220, 221, 222, 223
brainstem, 99, 100, 102, 103, 219
Breathe Right Strips®, 39
bruxism, 130
bupropion, 187
buttered cigarettes, 122

C

caffeine, 13, 15, 56, 111, 114, 116, 117, 126, 160, 189, 230
cancer, 167, 178
carbempazepine, 147
carbon dioxide, 52, 59, 99, 100, 103
Cardiologist, vii, 157
Cardiology, vi
catastrophication, 34
Cataplexy, 140
Catapress®, 134
CBT, 29
CCHS, 103
CDC, 54
Celexa®, 173, 186
centimeters of water, 71

Central Sleep Apnea, 52, 99, 102
Central Standard Time, 113
cerebrovascular accident, 165
cetirizine, 199
chamomile, 202
Charles Dickens, 59
Cheyne-Stokes Breathing, 101, 102, 156
chlorpheniramine, 199
chlorpromazine, 188
Chlortrimeton®, 199
choking, 52, 58, 61, 159
Chronic Bronchitis, 153
Chronic Interstitial Cystitis, 157
chronic pain, 149
Chronotherapy, 107
cimetidine, 160
circadian rhythm, 20, 105, 110, 179, 230, 231
citalopram, 173, 186
Claritin®, 199
clemastine, 199
clock genes, 105
clomipramine, 132, 187
clonazepam, 120, 122, 124, 135, 164, 196
clonidine, 134, 197, 198
codeine, 102, 122, 129, 193, 194
Cognitive Behavioral Therapy, 29
Complex Sleep Apnea, 102
computer screen, 11
Confusional Arousal, 119
Congenital Central Hypoventilation Syndrome, 103
Continuous Positive Airway Pressure, 69, 228
COPD, 153, 154, 235
cortex, 217
cough, 153
counseling, 27, 29, 167, 171, 172, 173, 174, 181, 206
CPAP, 40, 59, 60, 68, 69, 70, 71, 72, 73, 74, 75, 76, 77, 80, 81, 87, 91, 92, 93, 95, 96, 97, 101, 152, 154, 155, 238
CPAP titration study, 70, 96
CSA, 52

CVA, 165
Cymbalta®, 186

D

DA, 186
DDAVP®, 138
death rattle, 156
Decadron®, 200
Deep/Slow Wave Sleep, 3
deer tick, 168
Delayed Sleep Phase Syndrome,
    106, 109
delirium, 181
Deltasone®, 200
delusions, 175
Dementia, 135, 161, 163, 180, 237
Demerol®, 193
dentist, 41, 42, 76, 130
Depakote®, 188
Depression, 19, 21, 141, 146, 149,
    163, 166, 167, 168, 169, 170,
    171, 175, 177, 186, 213, 240,
    241, 243
desimpramine, 187
desmopressin, 138
desvenlafaxine, 186
Detrol®, 138
dexamethasone, 200
Dexedrine®, 145, 147, 175, 191
Dexilent®, 160
dexlansoprazole, 160
dextroamphetamine, 145, 147, 175,
    191
diagnostic sleep study, 63
dialysis, 158
diet, 77, 91, 160, 190
Dilantin®, 188
diphenhydramine, 195, 199
Ditropan®, 138
DME, 75, 95, 96
DNA, 105
domestic bliss, 38, 49
Domestic Travel, 111
dopamine, 127, 128, 129, 186, 196,
    220
doxepin, 33, 187

doxylamine, 195
drowsy driving, 60, 95
DSPS, 106
duloxetine, 186
durable medical equipment, 75, 95
Dymista®, 39

E

Ear, Nose, and Throat, 38, 68
EEG, 63, 165, 217, 239
Effexor®, 146, 174
EKG, 64
Elavil®, 134, 187, 195
electroacupuncture, 205
electrocardiogram, 64
electroencephalogram, 63
electromyography, 64
electrooculography, 64
Elmiron®, 158
email, 11
EMG, 64
Emphysema, 153
EMS, 203
Emsam®, 187
energy meridians, 204
ENT, vi, vii, 38, 39, 81, 92
Enuresis, 137, 234
EOG, 64
Eosinophilia-myalgia syndrome,
    203
Epworth Sleepiness Scale, 21, 22,
    27, 38, 57, 141
eReaders, 11
escitalopram, 186
esomeprazole, 160
eszipiclone, 32
exercise, 13, 29, 77, 134, 137, 151,
    205, 209, 223, 225
Exploding Head Syndrome, 132

F

Facebook®, 11
famotidine, 160
Farmer's Markets, 79
fast food, 78, 79
Fatal Familial Insomnia, 27

ferritin, 128, 164
fexofenadine, 199
Fibromyalgia, 150, 235, 236, 237, 243
First Night Effect, 62
Flonase®, 39
fluoxetine, 122, 134, 173, 186
fluphenazine, 188
fluvoxamine, 122, 173, 186
folk medicine, 201
foramen magnum, 99
full-face mask, 75

G

GABA, 221, 222
gabapentin, 129, 150, 194, 197
Gastroenterologist, 160
gastroesophageal reflux, 159
genioglossus advancement, 88
Geodon®, 188
GERD, 12, 151, 159, 160
glucose, 223
goggles, 116
Greenwich Mean Time, 113

H

Halcion®, 32, 196
Haldol®, 182, 188
hallucination, 118, 131, 176, 233
haloperidol, 182, 188
heart attack, 59, 69, 154
heart disease, 12, 28, 61, 71, 78
heart failure, 59, 69, 93, 99, 100, 138, 155, 156, 157
heartburn, 12, 159
Herbal Supplements, 202
herbs, 201
high blood pressure, 58
high resolution oximetry test, 66
HIV/AIDS, 168, 237, 238
HLA D15, 144
HLA DQB1*0602), 144
home sleep study, 65, 66
hormone replacement therapy, 178
Hospital Acquired Dementia, 181
hot flashes, 178

House, 124
HRT, 178
hydrocodone, 102, 193, 194
hydrocortisone, 200
Hyoid Advancement, 89
hyperpnea, 101
Hypersomnia, 147, 169, 177, 235
Hypnic Headaches, 163
Hypnic Jerks, 129
hypnogogic hallucination, 131, 141
hypnopompic hallucination, 131, 141, 233
Hypoglossal (tongue nerve) Stimulation Inspire, 87
hypopnea, 51, 64, 71, 72

I

ICSD-1, vi
ICU, 181
Idiopathic Hypersomnia, 147
Idiopathic Insomnia, 27
Idiopathic Pulmonary Fibrosis, 152
IL-1β, 167
Image Rehearsal Therapy, 134
imipramine, 137, 187
immune system, 167
Inderal®, 133, 197
Injection Snoreplasty, 48
innerspring mattresses, 9
Insomnia, 3, 13, 17, 18, 19, 21, 22, 23, 25, 26, 27, 28, 29, 34, 38, 149, 161, 164, 165, 167, 168, 169, 172, 174, 177, 180, 186, 204, 205, 206, 208, 213, 214, 225, 226, 235, 240, 246, 247, 248
Instagram®, 11
insurance, 38, 40, 42, 49, 69, 71, 73, 95, 108
Intensive Care Unit, 181
interleukin-1 beta, 167
Intermezzo®, 33
Internal Medicine, vi
International Travel, 112
Internist, vii
Invega®, 188

IPF, 152
iron, 128, 129, 158, 159, 164
iron binding capacity, 128
iron supplementation, 164
IRT, 134
isocarboxazid, 187

J

Jazz Pharmaceuticals, 146
JCAHO, 62
Jet Lag, 105, 110, 112, 114, 231
Jet Lag Prevention, 112
Joint Commission on Accreditation
of Healthcare Organizations, 62

K

Kava, 203
kegel exercises, 137
Keppra®, 188
Kidney failure, 158
Kleine Levin Syndrome, 123, 146
Klonopin®, 120, 122, 124, 135, 164,
196
KLS, 123, 146

L

Lamictal®, 188
lamotrigine, 188
lansoprazole, 160
Laser Assisted
Uvulopalatopharyngoplasty, 45
latex (solid foam) mattresses, 10
Latuda®, 188
LAUP, 45, 50
Law and Order, Special Victims
Unit, 124
levetiracetam, 188
Lexapro®, 186
Light Therapy, 108
lithium, 147, 163
Lithobid®, 147, 163
Lopressor®, 197
loratidine, 199
Lou Gehrig's disease, 162
L-tryptophan, 203

Luby's®, 180
Lunesta®, 32, 62, 195, 196
lurasidone, 188
Luvox®, 122, 173, 186
Lyme Disease, 168
Lyrica®, 129, 151, 194, 197

M

MAD, 41, 42, 50, 76
Maintenance of Wakefulness Test,
60, 96
Mandibular Advancement Device,
41, 42, 50, 76
Mania, 177
Marplan®, 187
mask, 69, 70, 71, 73, 74, 75, 76, 81,
95, 102, 162
mattress, 9
Maxillomandibular Advancement,
90
meditation, 29, 205, 206, 247
Melatonin, 105, 107, 108, 111, 112,
114, 116, 117, 151, 176, 195,
196, 201, 221, 222
memory foam mattresses, 10
Menopause, 178
meperidine, 193
methadone, 102, 193, 194
Methadose®, 102
methylphenidate, 145, 147, 175,
191, 241, 244
metoprolol, 197
Midline Tongue Reduction, 86
Minipress®, 134, 173, 197, 198
Mirapex®, 129, 159, 197
mirtazipine, 187
modafinil, 97, 116, 117, 145, 147,
166, 192, 229, 244
Morning Lark, 109
morphine, 193
MS, 166
MSLT, 144, 145
Multiple Sclerosis, 166
Multiple Sleep Latency Test, 144
MWT, 60, 96, 97

N

nap, 12, 14, 97, 116, 117, 144, 167, 176, 180, 199, 225
Narcolepsy, vi, 20, 65, 123, 131, 136, 140, 141, 144, 169, 192, 235
narcotics, 102, 149, 193
narcotized sleep, 149
Nasacort AQ®, 39
nasal congestion, 37, 38, 39, 43, 55, 61, 75, 82
Nasonex®, 39
National Institute for Health, 202
National Sleep Foundation, vi
neck circumference, 54
NES, 122
Neurology, vi
neurons, 216
Neurontin®, 129, 150, 194, 197
neurotransmitters, 219
Nexium®, 160
nicotine, 160, 192, 193
Night Eating Syndrome, 122
Night Owl, 106
night shift, 115
Night Terrors, 119
Nightmare Disorder, 133, 134, 173, 197
Nighttime Panic Disorder, 173
NIPPV, 162
non-dipper, 154
Non-Invasive Positive Pressure Ventilation, 162
non-REM sleep, 123, 125
Norco®, 102, 193, 194
norepinephrine/NE, 186
Norpramine®, 187
nortriptyline, 187
NPD, 173
NSF, 6
Nuvigil®, 97, 116, 117, 147, 166, 192

O

Obesity Hypoventilation Syndrome, 59

Obsessive Compulsive Disorder, 174
Obstructive Sleep Apnea, 41, 51, 52, 58, 59, 60, 61, 68, 80, 138, 152, 154, 226, 227, 228, 229, 230, 234, 239, 242
OCD, 174
OHS, 59
Oleptro®, 33, 187, 195
olopatadine, 39
omeprazole, 160
Ominvore's Dilemma, 79
optic nerve, 222
Oral Surgeon, 81, 92
Orgasms, 123
OSA, 40, 51, 54, 55, 60, 66, 68, 69, 73, 75, 76, 81, 83, 84, 85, 86, 87, 88, 89, 92, 97, 127, 152, 179
Otolaryngology – Head and Neck Surgery, vi
Overlap Syndrome, 153
oxybutynin, 138
oxycodone, 102, 193, 194
oxygen, 40, 52, 59, 64, 65, 66, 67, 68, 76, 99, 100, 101, 103, 153, 154
oxygen saturation, 52, 66

P

pain medicines, 193
Painful Bladder Syndrome, 157
Palatal Pillars, 46, 50
palate, 45, 50
paliperidone, 188
palpitations, 155
Pamelor®, 187
pantoprazole, 160
Paradoxical Insomnia, 27
Parkinson's Disease, 127, 135, 163, 238
Parnate®, 187
paroxetine, 122, 173, 186
Paroxysmal Nocturnal Dyspnea, 157
Patanase®, 39
Paxil®, 122, 173, 186
Pediatrician, vii, 171

Pediatrics, vi, 245
pentosan, 158
Percocet®, 102, 193, 194
Periodic Limb Movement Disorder, 127, 128, 169
Periodic Limb Movements of Sleep, 127
perphenazine, 188
phenytoin, 188
PHOX2B, 103
Pickwickian Syndrome, 59, 60
pillows, 9
pineal gland, 221
PLMD, 127, 128
PLMS, 127
PND, 157
Positional Therapy, 77
Postpartum Depression, 170
PPD, 170
pramipexole, 129, 159, 197, 233, 236
prazosin, 134, 173, 197, 198
prednisone, 200
pregabalin, 129, 151, 194, 197, 236
preoptic area, 221
Prevacid®, 160
Prilosec®, 160
Pristiq®, 186
Proair®, 198, 199
Progressive Deep Muscle Relaxation, 134
Progressive relaxation, 29
Prolixin®, 188
propranolol, 133, 197
proptriptyline, 187
prostate, 157
proton pump inhibitors, 160
Protonix®, 160
Provent®, 40, 50
Provigil®, 97, 116, 117, 145, 147, 166, 192
Prozac®, 122, 134, 173, 186
Psychophysiologic Insomnia, 26
psychotherapy, 151, 170, 173, 174
PTSD, 133, 134, 172, 173, 197, 241
Pulmonary Medicine, vi
Pulmonologist, vii

Q

Q'Nasl®, 39
Quackery, 208

R

rabeprozole, 160
Radiofrequency Palate Ablation, 47
Radiofrequency Tongue Base Reduction, 85
ramelteon, 161, 195, 196, 245
ranitidine, 160
rape, 124
RBD, 135, 163
Relaxation, 29, 202, 203, 205
Relaxation Therapy, 29
REM Behavior Disorder, 135, 163, 180, 234
REM Sleep, 3, 4, 5, 13, 25, 58, 64, 71, 77, 118, 121, 133, 134, 135, 136, 164, 173, 175, 176, 179, 196, 206, 234, 239
REM-A-TEE®, 77
Remeron®, 187
Requip®, 129, 159, 196
respiradone, 188
Restless Legs Syndrome, 127, 128, 129, 158, 164, 165, 168, 169, 180, 186, 196, 233, 238
Restoril®, 32, 196
risk for falling, 181
Risperidal®, 188
Ritalin®, 145, 175, 191
RLS, 128, 129, 158, 159, 164, 196
rohypnol, 146
ropinirole, 129, 159, 196, 244
Rozerem®, 161, 195, 196

S

safety, 116
Schizophrenia, 175, 176, 177, 240
SCN, 221
sedative, 26, 32, 62, 107, 116, 121, 124, 164, 166, 168, 172, 176, 185, 195, 242
seizures, 164, 187

selegine, 187
Sensory Sleep Starts, 129
Septoplasty, 43, 50, 81, 82
septum, 44, 82
serotonin/5HT, 186
sertraline, 173, 186
sex, 14, 123, 124
Sexomnia, 121, 123, 124, 125
sheets, 9
Shen Men, 204
Shiatsu, 204
Shift Work Syndrome, 106, 115
Silenor®, 33, 187
sleep anxiety, 27, 133
Sleep Challenge, 14
Sleep Diary, 23, 25, 27, 142
Sleep Drunkenness, 119
Sleep Hygiene, 8, 18, 26, 27, 29, 30,
    34, 161, 164, 166, 168, 176, 181,
    212
sleep lab, 61, 63, 65, 97, 123, 135,
    144, 202
Sleep Log, 23, 25, 27, 142
sleep mask, 113
Sleep Paralysis, 135, 136, 173, 233,
    234, 241
Sleep Related Eating Disorder, 121
Sleep Restriction, 30
Sleep Starts,, 129
Sleep State Misperception, 27, 174
Sleep Talking, 121
Sleep Violence, 121, 125, 126
Sleep walking, 120
Sleeping pills, 194
snore, 19, 28, 37, 38, 46, 53, 212
snoring, iii, 36, 37, 38, 39, 40, 41,
    42, 43, 44, 45, 46, 47, 48, 49, 51,
    53, 54, 56, 58, 61, 65, 66, 70, 81,
    82, 83, 84, 85, 87, 88, 89, 90,
    141, 180, 208, 209, 210, 211,
    212, 226, 227
sodium oxybate, 145, 146
Solucortef®, 200
Somnambulism, 120
Somniloquy, 121
Sonata®, 32
sotalol, 197

Split Night Sleep Study, 71
Split Night Study, 71
SRED, 121, 122
SSRI, 173
Stage 1 Sleep, 3, 25
Stage 2 Sleep, 3
Stage 3 Sleep, 3, 25, 119, 179
Stanford University, vi
Starbucks®, 13
Stiff Man Syndrome, 150
stimulant, 13, 15, 117, 174, 175,
    189, 192
Stimulus Control, 30
stroke, 59, 69, 102, 135, 165, 239
Substance S, 223
Sundowning, 181
suprachiasmatic nucleus, 221
Surmontil®, 187
suvorexant, 33, 195, 196, 226, 246

T

tagamet®, 160
Tai Chi Chih, 205
TAM, 203
Tavist®, 199
Tegretol®, 147, 187
temazepam, 32, 196
temporomandibular joint, 76
texting, 11
thalamus, 219
The International Classification of
    Sleep Disorders, vi
Theodur®, 198
theophylline, 198
therapeutic light bank, 116
Theravent®, 40
Thorazine®, 188
TMJ, 42, 76, 130
TNF-α, 167
Tofranil®, 137, 187
tolterodine, 138
Tonsillectomy, 44, 85
tonsils, 44
Topamax®, 122, 188
topiramate, 122, 132, 188
Toprax®, 132

Tracheotomy, 91
Traditional Asian Medicine, 203
tramadol, 193
tranylcypromine, 187
trazadone, 33, 187
tremors, 163
triazolam, 32, 196
Trilafon®, 188
trimipramine, 187
Tumblr®, 11
tumor necrosis factor-alpha, 167
Turbinate Reduction, 43, 81, 82
turbinates, 44, 82
Type 2 Diabetes, 12

U

Ultram®, 193
Uniphyl®, 198
Unisom®, 195
UPPP, 84
urethra, 157
Urologist, 157
Uvulopalatopharyngoplasty, 84

V

Valerian, 202
valproic acid, 188
venlafaxine, 146, 174
Vicodin®, 102, 193, 194
Vivactil®, 187

W

Wakefulness Promoters, 192
wake-promoter, 97
Waterbeds,, 10
weight, 37, 53, 54, 59, 60, 61, 68,
    77, 78, 80, 96, 170
weight loss, 78
Wellbutrin®, 187
witnessing sleep, 206

X

Xyrem®, 145, 146

Y

yoga, 206

Z

zaleplon, 32
Zantac®, 160
Zegerid®, 160
ziprasidone, 188
Zoloft®, 173, 186
zolpidem, 32, 33, 62, 113, 114, 151,
    164, 195, 196
zolpidem tartrate, 33, 195
Zyrtec®, 199
ZZoma®, 77

About the Author

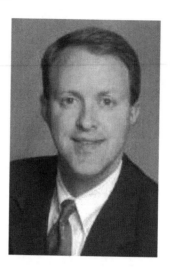

Mark T. Brown, MD, FACS, graduated magna cum laude from Texas Christian University with a Bachelors of Science in Biology. He completed his doctorate of medicine at Baylor College of Medicine and his residency in Otolaryngology – Head and Neck Surgery (Ear, Nose, and Throat to the rest of us) and fellowship in Head and Neck Surgical Reconstruction at The Massachusetts Eye and Ear Infirmary, a teaching hospital of Harvard Medical School.

After serving an appointment as an Assistant Professor of Otolaryngology at Johns Hopkins School of Medicine, he entered private practice in Austin, TX. He has enjoyed a twenty-plus year career in healthcare. His practice in Austin, Great Hills ENT (greathillsent.com), is a nationally (JHACO) accredited sleep center.

Dr. Brown pursued his specialty in Sleep Medicine after he began his clinical practice. He is board certified in both Sleep Medicine and Otolaryngology.

His passion to educate patients led him to share his expertise and experiences in "Smarter Sleep". He hopes to sleep better himself, now that he has published this book!

Made in the USA
San Bernardino, CA
13 July 2015